Breastfeeding Sucks

What to Do When Your
Mammaries Make You Miserable

Joanne Kimes,
author of *Pregnancy Sucks*

Technical Review by Suzanne Fredregill,
coauthor of *The Everything® Breastfeeding Book*

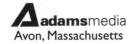
Adamsmedia
Avon, Massachusetts

To my daughter, Emily. You make each day so much
better just by being in it. I love you to pieces.

Published by
Adams Media, an F+W Publications Company
57 Littlefield Street, Avon, MA 02322 U.S.A.
www.adamsmedia.com

ISBN-10: 1-59337-628-6
ISBN-13: 978-1-59337-628-4
Printed in Canada.

J I H G F E D C B A

Library of Congress Cataloging-in-Publication Data
Kimes, Joanne.
Breastfeeding sucks / Joanne Kimes.
p.   cm.
ISBN-13: 978-1-59337-628-4 (pbk.)
ISBN-10: 1-59337-628-6 (pbk.)
1. Breastfeeding. I. Title.
RJ216.K474 2007
649'.33—dc22
                                2007015785

This publication is designed to provide accurate and authoritative
information with regard to the subject matter covered. It is sold with
the understanding that the publisher is not engaged in rendering professional medical advice. If assistance is required, the services of a com-
petent medical professional should be sought. The views expressed are
solely those of the author.
— From a *Declaration of Principles* jointly adopted by a Committee of the
American Bar Association and a Committee of Publishers and Associations

Many of the designations used by manufacturers and sellers to distin-
guish their product are claimed as trademarks. Where those designations appear in this book and Adams Media was aware of a trademark
claim, the designations have been printed with initial capital letters.

This book is available at quantity discounts for bulk purchases.
For information, please call 1-800-289-0963.

contents

Chapter 3
"Nursing" Your Wounds 69

Chapter 4
Feeding Frustrations. 99

Acknowledgments

Breastfeeding isn't easy. Neither is writing about it. That's because there are so many different experiences and situations that come into play that can affect its success. But thanks to the dozens of lovely lactaters who shared their tales of woe, I feel all the breastfeeding bases have been covered. A giant thanks to the following women who were especially helpful: Allison Shallert, Lizzy Bauer, Megan Town, Sarah Redmond, Kate Epstein, and Marjorie Praytor-Costner.

Even though they didn't suckle any babies on their bosoms, a big thank you goes out as well to my agent, Jeff Herman, and my editors, Jennifer Kushnier and Meredith O'Hayre. And thanks of course to my husband, Jeff Kimes, for being as supportive as one of my enormous nursing bras. I love you.

Chapter 1

Got Breast Milk?

Breastfeeding is a natural bodily function performed by every mammal in the animal kingdom. Only in the human animal is it as controversial as gay marriage. Everyone has an opinion on what's the easiest way to do it, what products to have on hand to get it done, and how long you need to partake in the experience. And everyone is quite generous with their opinions, not unlike how they were during your pregnancy when perfect strangers would warn you about miscarriages, stretch marks, and pooping on the delivery room table.

But unlike the political aspects of gay marriage, breastfeeding is a very personal experience. Because of this, only you can decide what's best for you—although your mother-in-law will most certainly chime in on the topic. You need to factor in all the various elements so you can make an informed decision. There is so much information on the topic that writers like me have devoted entire books to the breastfeeding experience, all in an attempt to inform, enlighten, and okay, make a few bucks as well. (Hey, I have my own kid to put through college!)

Whether or not you want to breastfeed is a big decision. Fortunately, your nine-month stint of pregnancy has prepared you for making such big decisions. You had to decide if you wanted to know the sex of the baby before it was born. You had to decide on a name. And you had to decide if you wanted an epidural during delivery, although for me that was a no-brainer since I think pain-killers are the next best thing to bleach pens.

To make your decision even easier, and to help guide you along the path once your decision has been made, I'll take you through every aspect of breastfeeding, from colostrum through clogged ducts, and I'll do so in baby steps. It's like pressing the "Easy" button on lactation. Lord knows, you have enough stress to deal with already in your life, and anything to reduce it is a good thing. You don't need to be overwhelmed by another aspect of parenthood right now. Breastfeeding is like nothing you've ever experienced before; the basic idea that milk will soon start spewing from your breasts is a pretty freaky thought. It's like blowing your nose and having Skittles fly out.

While I'm sure many of you are already nursing, I'll bet a vat of nipple cream that many more of you are still pregnant and reading ahead, as you know that your leisure hours will be severely limited once your baby makes his appearance. (By the way, I'm going to refer to all babies as "he." That's not because I'm partial to boys—it's because my *S* key tends to stick, and anything that reduces my stress level is a good thing.) Because of the variation in levels of experience, we'll start at the very beginning of the lactating journey and work our way out from there. If you've already started nursing, just jump right in whenever you'd like. So let's get to it before your desire to breastfeed fades or your contractions begin!

A Shove in the Right Direction

Maybe you're on the fence about whether breastfeeding is right for you. You've heard the horror stories. You've been warned about the pain. And you've seen the size of the nursing bras. Whether or not you want to nurse is a big decision, and you probably have a hard enough time deciding between paper and plastic. If this is the case, I'll help you do what anyone faced with a big decision should do, whether it be to marry someone or to choose which flavor ice cream to eat. It's time to make a list.

In order to help you make the decision of whether breastfeeding is right for you and to help push you over the fence, I've compiled a list of the good, the bad, and the ugly sides of nursing so that you can make an informed decision.

The Good

1. **Breast milk is the beverage of choice for your baby.** It's the Dom Perignon of the diaper set. Not only does it taste delicious to their tender palates, but it's easy to digest and chock-full of disease-fighting agents that help your little one stay well. Studies show that a breastfed baby is less likely to, suffer from ear infections, diarrhea, colic, and bacterial infections. It's also been claimed that breastfeeding lowers the risk of contracting SIDS, meningitis, type

I diabetes, childhood lymphomas, allergies, asthma, and leukemia. If you ask me, we should never stop drinking the stuff and should add it to our morning cereal.

2. **Breastfeeding is better for the mother's health as well.** Studies have shown that women who breastfeed have a lower risk of developing ovarian cancer and premenopausal breast cancer. Besides, having your baby nurse causes your uterus to contract after delivery like a Shrinky Dink. And that's important since at that point, your poor organ looks like it's been put through a taffy pull.

3. **Nursing is a whole lot cheaper than formula.** In fact, if you breastfeed for a year, you could save between $900 and $4,700! That's enough to put your kid through eight whole days of private school!

4. **Breastfeeding can help you bond with your baby.** Don't worry if you don't bond with your kid when he's fresh from the chute. It's a fallacy that when women give birth, they always look at their newborns and are automatically bonded for a lifetime. Sometimes all you feel is incredible relief that he's finally out and you're not in any

more pain. But once you start nursing, the process does tend to connect you with your child like nothing else in life ever will.

5. **You'll have more free time.** There's nothing easier than whipping out a boob whenever your baby's tummy starts a-rumbling. Sure, you may need to nurse more often; breast milk is more easily digested, so babies eat more often than they would with formula. But when you factor in the time it takes to run to Costco every two weeks to load up on formula, sterilize the nipples and bottles, and prepare and warm the formula, you still come out way ahead.

6. **You'll have less stress when you're on the go.** Getting out of your house with a kid involves more packing than a month-long trip to Honduras. But the chore becomes much made doable when you don't have to lug around bottles, formula packets, water bottles, sterilizers, and bottle warmers.

7. **If you're going back to work and will pump so that you can continue to feed your baby mother's milk, chances are you'll need to take off fewer days from work.** That's because breast milk is shown

to keep your baby healthier than if you feed him formula.

8. **You can eat more!** A nursing mother needs about 500 extra calories per day in order to produce all that milk! Is there any better reason to nurse? I think not.

The Bad

1. You're shy and don't want to pull a "Janet Jackson" in front of a crowd whenever it's feeding time.

2. **You're afraid of how much nursing will hurt.** After suffering through the pains and discomforts of pregnancy, you're maxed out for a lifetime . . . and you haven't even gone into labor yet!

3. **No matter how much you may want him to, your husband will never be able to lactate, and that means he won't be able to help out with midnight feedings (unless you pump bottles).** Men. They have less body fat, more upper body strength, and will never have to deal with cracked nipples. Thank goodness they go bald.

4. **You're afraid that after you're done breast-feeding, your breasts will sag.** If that's your fear, relax. Studies have shown that nursing isn't to blame for saggy breasts. Heredity is the first and most important factor in sagging. Further, pregnancy with all the hormones and increased breast tissue, makes your boobs sag like Tiffani Amber Thiessen's career. Feel better?

5. **Breast milk doesn't have the "stick-to-your-ribs" quality that formula does, so a breastfed baby usually needs more feedings than one who's given formula.**

6. **You've read that if you nurse, the hormones can make sex painful.** Unlike the myth of sagging, this one is actually true. If you choose to breastfeed, intercourse can be uncomfortable, at least for awhile. Lubricants help, as does time. After awhile your body will adjust but even then, you still won't like sex. That's not because it will hurt but because you'll be too tired to enjoy it.

The Ugly

1. **The poopy diapers of breastfed babes are sweeter-smelling than the poopy diapers of formula-fed ones.** Considering

the enormous amount of poopy diapers that you'll be changing, this fact alone should warrant you giving breastfeeding a try.

Are Your Breasts Worthy?

Even if you think that breast milk is better, there may be several reasons why you feel it's not the right choice for you. For one, you may have a serious health condition like TB or hepatitis B, or one that's not as serious but that still requires the use of medication that could be passed on to your baby through your breast milk. It's perfectly understandable if these or any other medical concerns are making you say no to nursing. At the same time, there are several other conditions that you may think are a problem but that are, in truth, no problem at all.

Having inverted or flat nipples is one major concern. True, while it might be more challenging to get your baby to latch on to a nipple that's gone into hiding, it certainly isn't impossible. But it will require a bit more work and the help from a few modern-day miracles like nipple shields and breast pumps. (See "Flat or Inverted Nipples" on page 75 for more details.)

"I had my breasts reduced in my young twenties, and ten years later I had my first child. I was worried that I wouldn't make enough milk, but just the opposite happened. I had so much milk that my boobs would literally squirt milk across the room."

—Lori

Having breast implants is another popular concern. Today, breast implants are as socially acceptable as $3 cups of coffee. With the increased amount of breast augmentations comes the increased amount of worry that these enhanced mammary glands won't be able to do what they were put on the planet to do: produce milk. If you've had a breast enlargement and are concerned about this aspect, relax. Since most implants are placed behind the breast tissue, most breasts should still be able to produce milk. There is a potentially valid concern about how much milk they will actually produce, since the surgery may impede their production, but you'll never know until you try. Worse comes to worse, you may need to supplement with formula after you nurse.

Conversely, women who have undergone breast reduction surgery may worry that their minimized breasts won't be up for the task either. Even though large breasts are as much a fashion statement these days as low-rise jeans, some women actually go under the knife to make their breasts smaller. Now that these women are pregnant, they worry that their smaller breasts may not be up to the enormous demand of milk production. Plus, they may be pissed that they spent thousands of dollars to reduce what Mother Nature is now enhancing. Whether or not a reduced breast can produce milk depends on the type of surgery. If the nipple was removed and relocated as a result of reduction, you may not be able to produce milk.

If you have a pierced nipple, you may be concerned about nursing as well. Why oh why anyone would want to stick a needle through one of the most sensitive areas of her body is beyond me, but I'll try to remain nonjudgmental. Whatever these people want to do is fine by me. But if you were brave/crazy enough to have your nipple pierced, there are a couple of things you should know. First, you may have more discomfort than other women because nipple piercing and the scarring it creates may increase the sensitivity of the nipple. Although increased sensitivity may have been the effect you were after when you had it done, now it's coming back to bite where it counts. You may also experience more leakage from a pierced nipple than one that remains intact. And finally, you must always remove the nipple ring prior to nursing to keep it from falling out and choking your baby. I know that sounds obvious, but hey, you went ahead and stuck a needle through your nipple, so I just want to make sure that this point is perfectly clear.

Those of you with small breasts may have breastfeeding concerns as well. It's natural to think that the smaller the breast, the less likely it will perform well compared with its oversized counterparts. That's because we live in a society where bigger is thought to be better. SUVs are more desirable than subcompacts. Big Gulps are better than a can of soda. And multiplex theaters are superior to single screens, if you can even find a single-screen theater anymore. But I disagree, and so does Mother Nature. Since bigger breasts simply contain more fat (or silicone or saline for that matter) than small ones, having small boobies does not affect your ability to produce milk. It may detract from their ability to fill out a halter top, perhaps, but not to produce milk.

And finally, women with hairy nipples may have specific concerns as well. I realize that having hair on your breasts may sound odd, but for women with darker complexions or for those who have been affected by excess hair growth during pregnancy, the concern is real. But don't worry, be happy! Any extra hair around your nipple area will in no way harm your baby. Many of us women have had our mouths in hairy places, and we are still living full and healthy lives.

As you can see, there are many reasons to fear that your breasts may not be worthy of nursing. But like my dad always says, "You can't catch any fish unless you go fishing." Okay, I may need to reword that a bit to ring true in this case, so here goes: "You can't nurse any young unless you start lactating." Therefore, unless your doctor advises you to pass on nursing because it could harm either you or your baby, why not give it a try and see what happens? Even if you have a pierced, augmented, hairy breast with an inverted nipple, you should still be good to go!

Under Pressure

As much as I encourage any able-bodied and able-boobied woman to give nursing a go, you shouldn't feel pressure from me, or anyone else for that matter, to breastfeed if it isn't something that you want to do. Nursing is the first in a long line of parental decisions that you will be making, and you need to have the inner strength to believe in your convictions. Whether it be how you discipline your child, what immunizations you want him to have, or how goofily you want to dress him for his school picture, feel confident that the decision you make is the right one for you.

But be prepared. If you choose not to nurse, you may get some flack from society. Nursing mothers may look at you in a judgmental manner. You may get sneers from your relatives as well. Onlookers can make you feel like you're the worst mother in the world if you feed your baby anything other than breast milk. Right now, nursing is all the rage. A couple of generations ago, it was the exception, and doing so would have gotten you stares as well. Like hem lengths, the popularity of nursing keeps changing.

But that doesn't mean that nursing moms don't get stares either. In fact, they get plenty of them. As much as society pressures you into nursing, other people are also the first ones who make you feel uncomfortable when you do it in public. Some find this behavior very offensive and think of it as being in the same vein as a Vegas strip act.

So whether you decide to nurse, or not to nurse, feel confident about your decision. Try not

to care what other people think about your decisions, whether it be about breastfeeding or that
hokey sailor outfit you put your kid in for his
yearly photo. You're the parent. You make the
decisions. And if anyone has a problem with it,
just send that person to bed without any supper!

Lactation Lingo

Learning something new often entails decipher-
ing a brand-new language. If you take up cooking, you'll need to become familiar with words
like sauté and chiffonade. If scrapbooking's your
thing, it's phrases like, "I can't believe you're
charging so much for this small piece of crap!"
Breastfeeding is no exception to this rule, and it
too comes with its own vernacular. Here are some
key terms to know before you enter the business
of breastfeeding:

Nipple: This is the dense pointy part of your
breasts that pops up out like a turkey timer.

Areola: The darker pigmented skin that surrounds
the nipple. If you've noticed during pregnancy,
your areola has become much darker in color and

much larger in size. Studies show that the reason for this transformation is so that your colorblind newborn can easily locate it when it's time for a feeding. I thought that was interesting.

Colostrum: Think of this as starter milk. It's what your breasts produce while you're pregnant and during the first days after your baby is born. It's very nutritious and high in calories. It's the trail mix of breast milk, if you will.

Foremilk: Once your milk comes in, it makes up the majority of your milk supply and represents about 90 percent of the type of breast milk that your baby will consume.

Hindmilk: The thicker and denser milk that comes at the end of your milk supply on each breast. It's like that thick blob of syrup that collects at the bottom of a glass of chocolate milk.

Let down: The process of getting your milk to flow from your ducts down to your nipple. This term can have double meaning to a new mommy because it also refers to how she feels once those baby blues have set in.

Latch on: It's the way a baby adheres to his mother's breast. If done incorrectly, it's the thing that's responsible for all the screaming.

Prep Work

If after weighing all the pros and cons you decide to give breastfeeding a spin, you're in luck. Unlike most other activities you want to indulge in, getting ready to breastfeed requires no phone calls, no to-do lists, and no errands. In fact, you don't have to do a thing except sit back and let Mother Nature do all the work for you. Your body is a one-stop-shop when it comes to milk production, and it can take care of all the details for you. I was amazed by how my body could effortlessly produce milk when it had so much trouble learning the simple act of rubbing my belly with one hand and patting my head with the other.

Although there isn't anything you need to do in order to produce the breast milk itself, there is something you can do to make nursing a bit easier if you have flat or inverted nipples. You can use your last month of pregnancy to help them

stand up and be counted for. Ask your obste-
trician if it's okay to use a breast shell to help
pop out your nipples (breast shells are available
at most pharmacies and baby stores). Or, if you
prefer, you can use your fingers to help squeeze
them out, just like you would a blackhead. Just
place your index fingers on the opposite sides of
the end of your areola and pull outward. Do this
several times a day, but make sure that you use
only gentle stimulation. (Don't tug or squeeze, as
this can cause tissue damage.)

You should know that there's an old wives'
tale floating around that before you deliver,
you'll need to toughen up your nipples to prepare them to be sucked on. I'm not sure how
this rumor got started. Maybe it's because the
ninth month of pregnancy is so nerve-wracking
that you'll neurotically do anything you can to
pass the time. But the last thing your tender
nipples need is to be rubbed until they're as
tough as a supreme court justice. The truth is
that your nipples are ready to breastfeed just
the way they are. They don't need to be rubbed
with washcloths or exposed to air. I know this
will give you even fewer things to do during
the ninth month, but perhaps you can use the
extra time to try to master that rubbing-your-

belly-while-patting-your-head thing. It really does present quite a challenge.

Boobie Prize

Although you don't have to pay for breast milk, you do have to pay for the dozens of items that are designed to help the process along. True, women have been breastfeeding long before the creation of Target and Babies "R" Us, but hey, your boobs have to go through quite an ordeal, so you really should get them a few thank-you gifts. Of course, like many other baby items on your list, from hooded towels to diaper-wipe warmers, you could survive without them, but why should you? Your breasts deserve the very best! So here are a few must-haves that all the "in" breasts are wearing:

Boppy: This is a big comfy pillow shaped like the letter C. Just wrap it around your waist like an oversized belt, sit down, and set your baby on top of it to nurse. Using a Boppy brings your baby up to a more comfortable feeding level so that you don't have to scrunch or strain your neck. Later, as your baby grows and learns how to sit up, you can place him inside the Boppy. It will support his back so he doesn't flop all over like a sock puppet. A Boppy is not only practical, but it comes in dozens of pastel colors and animal prints to match any nursery decor.

My Brest Friend: This is an alternative to the Boppy. If you're having trouble getting your baby to latch on correctly, this is an excellent product to have.

Lanolin cream: This very dense lotion is derived from sheep's wool and is great to prevent and relieve dry, cracked nipples, if you're not allergic to wool. Keep in mind that the best cure for cracked nipples is breast milk, which you simply rub on the wound. Mother Nature thinks of everything!

Breast pads: These are soft, absorbent pads to put inside of your bra. They absorb leaks so it doesn't look like your boobs are sweating. Breast pads come in various types, such as disposable, plastic coated, and some that even have lanolin built right in.

Breast pump: Even if you're a stay-at-home mom, you may want a breast pump. Not only can it relieve engorgement, but you can pump and store bottles so that Daddy can help with feedings, or so that you can go to the market and linger over nutritional labels. Believe me, once you have a baby, you'll realize how relaxing and enjoyable a supermarket is when you don't have a screaming kid with you.

Plastic storage bags for pumped milk: Once you pump the milk, you gotta have something to put it in. That's why manufacturers have created overpriced plastic freezer bags that have measurements written on the side to keep track of how many ounces you've pumped.

Bottle warmer: Now that you've pumped your milk and stored it in convenient bags, you need a way to warm it up back up again. You can't do it in a microwave because that method can create hot spots. Sure, you could do it on the stove in some warm water, but why should you when you can buy an electric gizmo to do the job for you? They even make bottle warmers in travel size so you can warm up a bottle while you're on the go. (Entrepreneurs think of everything, too.)

Sterilizer: If this is your second kid, you'll simply give your bottles and pacifiers a quick rinse before using them. (If it's your third, you'll just blow off the germs.) But for your first baby, you'll want a sterilizer that cleans them so well that you could use them during open-heart surgery.

Baby sling: Technically, a sling won't help you with milk production or in the effort to ease sore nipples. But it's a great place to nurse your baby, especially when you need to use your hands to do other things. The sling is so relaxing and snug, it's like a La-Z-Boy for newborns.

Good chair and footstool: You can certainly nurse while sitting in any chair (after your stitches heal, of course), but when it comes to nursing our wee little lads and lassies, we conjure up romantic images of doing so in an antique rocker or sleek glider. My advice? Don't spend a lot of money on these. You won't be using it for that long a time, and soon, you'll want it out of the room to provide more play space. Whatever chair you decide on, get a foot stool as well. Your neck will thank you.

Let's Get This Pumping Started!

What new mom doesn't look at a metallic, milk-sucking breast pump and get scared out of her mind? These contraptions look and sound so downright terrifying that some producer would be wise to make a horror movie about them, entitled *I Know What You Pumped Last Summer*. But as scary as a breast pump can be, trust me when I say it'll soon become your most productive appliance, next to your coffeemaker. It can help out with a multitude of problems.

A breast pump is not only vital if you're returning to work and want to continue feeding your baby breast milk, it can also help out with painful nursing ailments like engorgement and breast clogs. In addition, having a pump allows you to make a stockpile of bottles and store them in the freezer for up to six months, thus allowing you and your husband to go off on a romantic weekend getaway (or more likely, run out for a quick McMeal whenever you're able to find a good sitter).

If you're still pregnant, you won't be using a breast pump anytime soon unless you're looking for an alternative way to squeeze fresh orange juice, so for now, we'll focus on which pump to choose. (If you're looking for help using a pump, see "Pumping Problems" on page 116.) Buying a breast pump can be confusing. There are many different manufacturers and many different styles to chose from. But in sum, they can be broken down into three different types. To simplify matters, here's the 4-1-1 on the P-U-M-P:

Manual pump: This affordable style is operated by the power of your hand or foot. It isn't necessarily the easiest way to pump, but it can be the quickest way to get back into shape since it's so physically taxing to use! It's good if you only need to express a little bit of milk to relieve engorgement or to make the occasional bottle. The downfall of the manual pump is that you can only pump one breast at a time, and it's bad for anyone who's prone to carpal tunnel syndrome or just suffering from sheer fatigue.

Handheld battery-operated pump: This is basically a manual pump without the manual part since it operates on batteries. Sure, it does give your arm or leg muscles a break, but it still only pumps one breast at a time and is usually much slower than an electric pump. Again, it's only good for occasional pumping since the motor isn't very strong.

Electric pump: This is the Ferrari of the pumping world. The various models are strong and sturdy and look quite impressive. They're designed for fast, double pumping so that your breasts get in and out of there as quickly as possible. You can buy electric pumps in baby shops and discount stores, but if you want to go for the top of the line, get one that's hospital grade. (These can be rented, if you prefer, because the cost of buying one is usually quite high.) Electric pumps are by far the most expensive of all pumps, but if you plan to pump long and often, one will certainly make your life easier. Plus, if you plan on having more than one child, you can amortize the expense, thus rationalizing the price better. We women always need a way to rationalize a big purchase.

Like most things in life, you get what you pay for (in my experience true of all things except mascara, since I find the drugstore brands work just as well as their expensive department-store counterparts). Breast pumps are like automobiles that come with many options. The less you pay, the less you get. There's speed control, suction control, automatic cycling, two-phase pumps, breast shield design, and power source options. Tell the salesperson about your pumping plans so you can get the best options for your needs.

When you use your breast pump for the first time, you'll envision yourself a heifer at a dairy farm. A terrorized heifer, nonetheless, since attaching your tender breasts to a powerful metal contraption fills your body with fear and your head full of that *Chucky* horror-movie theme music. Your body will tremble as your round full breasts are contorted into cone-shaped points. Once you turn the machine on (to the lowest possible setting), you'll relax as you realize there is no pain.

"I couldn't believe how expensive breast pumps were, so I thought it best to borrow my neighbor's manual pump. I figured, how hard could it be to pump when milk would leak out without even trying? Turns out, it's damn hard to get the milk out when you want it to, and far too easy when you're wearing a silk blouse."

—Anna

Just gentle tugging. You can experiment if you'd like, but if you feel any pain or discomfort, you should immediately put the machine on a lower setting. Over time, using a pump won't be at all scary; for now, just cover your ears and keep your eyes closed.

Booby Traps, aka Nursing Bras

You may have heard through the pregnancy grapevine that you should wait until you deliver your baby before you buy your nursing bras. That's because, as big as your bosoombas are now, they're only a coming attraction compared with the enormity that they'll become once your milk comes in. Although it's true that your breasts can grow as much as two cup sizes after the birth of your baby, I still suggest that you buy your nursing bras during your last month of pregnancy. And I think this for one very good reason: Once your baby is born, you'll be up to your bloodshot, exhausted eyeballs coping with your new life, your new baby, and the dizzying array of visitors who will descend upon your home in need of constant entertainment and food. The last thing you'll want to do is deal with a crowded mall to shop for undergarments.

So enjoy the calm before the storm, and go to a store that specializes in nursing bras. Then, find a salesperson who knows what she's doing who can measure you, estimate how much you may grow, and educate you on the wonderful world of nursing bras—a world that's filled with many different sizes and styles to choose from. There are the kinds that snap from the inner corners, ones that snap from the top, and the ones that are built right into clothing. And even though your boobs are still growing, I urge you to get a tran-sition bra now. Transitional bras are like clown cars. They can accommodate your breasts at the size they are now *and* at the enormous size they will become once your milk comes in.

Nursing bras can be expensive, but they're well worth the price. If you must, pass up those classi-cal music tapes that promise to raise your baby's IQ, and buy more bras that promise to raise your heavy hooters instead. Nursing bras are built like a semi to support your extra-wide load.

In terms of how many bras to buy, might I sug-gest three: one to wear, one for your drawer, and one for the laundry. Because milk leakage can be a problem the first few months of nursing, they will need to be washed frequently. Also, because you'll no doubt be wearing them morning, noon, and night to support your "girls," you'll never want to be without this constant source of support.

Yes, all in all, nursing bras are a must-have for the lactation set. Not only are they attractive so you can hold your head high, they're built so well that they'll hold your breasts even higher. Plus you can even use them after you've weaned your baby since they make wonderful covers for your BBQ or SUV.

Chapter 2

Newborns Suck-le

You did it! You gave birth. Whether you had a vaginal birth or were cracked open like a box of Cracker Jack to get to the hidden prize, you got that baby out of you, and you feel fantastic! After all those months of waiting, you can finally hold your precious miracle, gaze into his gorgeous eyes, and more important, sleep on your stomach once again! Congratulations and hooray for you!

And what a glorious baby he is! He has ten sweet fingers and ten delicious toes and, oddly enough, a hearty appetite as well. Who knew that traveling down a five-inch birth canal could bring on such strong hunger pains? It's as if your kid decided to pull over and take a Pilates class along the way. Whatever the reason, you'll find that not long after your kid pops out, it's feeding time!

The timing, of course, could not be worse. Here it is, just minutes after you've gone through the most painful, horrific, and labor intensive ordeal of your life, and you can't even kick back with a tabloid magazine. Instead, you have to deny your own needs for those of your child. Welcome, my friend, to the world of parenthood, where you'll be residing for the next eighteen fun-filled years!

Yes, this is only the first in a long list of situations that you'll be faced with, in which your baby's needs must come before your own. You won't be able to sleep through the night because your kid will need to eat every few hours. You won't be able to pee when the urge hits you because your baby will cry whenever you leave the room. And you won't be able to watch reruns of *Sex and the City* at the end of a long day because your baby will want to watch that danged purple dinosaur for the billionth time that day. It's enough to make you rip the head off that prehistoric beast.

But we're getting ahead of ourselves. For now, let's all take a deep cleansing breath and stick to the issue at hand: nursing. Yes, your kid is finally out in the world, and it's time to put all your obsessive baby-book reading to the test! Crank up those boobies because your life as a dairy queen has officially begun!

Milk Made

I've always been interested in medicine and love watching television shows like *ER* and *Grey's Anatomy* (although I admit my main interest in that show is Dr. McDreamy). Even though I've learned the basics about the inner workings of my body, I was completely mystified when it came to understanding how my body produced milk. Not once in any show did a woman have trouble with her milk-making gland. And never did one have to be rushed into surgery for an immediate the-organ-that-makes-milk-ectomy. If you're as baffled as I was about the makings of this delicious beverage, allow me to fill you in on the basics.

To being with, unlike the pancreas, which is responsible for producing bile, or bone marrow, whose responsibility is to produce blood cells (see, I really do watch those shows), there is no single organ that makes milk. Breast milk is actually formed in small groups of cells called alveoli that are located inside your breast tissue. These alveoli are surrounded by fat and connective tissue, which protects them like bubble wrap. Once the milk is produced, it then travels down the milk ducts and is stored behind your areola. Then, your baby starts sucking on your areola, and the milk is released through the holes in your nipples. Yes, I did say "holes." Surprise, surprise, there isn't just one hole in your nipple, as you may have thought. Instead, a nipple has many tiny holes and somewhat resembles a spaghetti strainer.

Now that we've discussed how the milk is made, let's go over the several different varieties of milk that your dairy farm produces. In the beginning, there is colostrum. As early as your forth month of pregnancy, you may have noticed a thick yellowish substance leaking from your nipples. Or, if you neurotically wore a bra every minute of the day and night in hopes of avoiding saggy breasts like I did, you may have noticed some flakiness around the nipple area. Yes, even early on in pregnancy, milk production had begun, which explains why your breasts have doubled in bulk like warm bread dough.

Colostrum is much richer than breast milk. It's loaded with protein, antibodies, vitamins, and minerals and is buttery yellow in color (a lovely shade to brighten up a dark room). In addition to its nutrients, colostrum also has a similar effect to that first cup of morning coffee: It helps your baby get rid of his first meconium poop (a tar-colored discharge that I don't believe comple-ments any room in the house).

After a few days of nursing, your colostrum goes bye-bye and is replaced with something called *transitional milk.* Very thin and white in color, transitional milk is the Kate Bosworth of breast milk. It should only take a day or two to come in, but you'll know it has arrived when your cleavage becomes the size of Cleveland.

After several days of these milk warm-up acts, the headliner finally makes its grand entrance. Breast milk. It's the perfect food for your child, given that it comes complete with everything he needs to stay healthy. At first, you may be sur-prised by the appearance of breast milk, which looks quite different from any milk you've seen in the past. It's quite watery, because it contains less fat than cow's milk, and is a bit bluish in color. When you try it, you'll notice that it tastes different than cow's milk, too. It has a sweet yet subtle hint of cantaloupe flavor. Now don't bother telling me that you're not going to try it. We all do. We ate paste as a kid, and perhaps a couple of dog biscuits on a dare, and we're all going to try this, too. It's one of the secrets of mommy-dom, like how much your vulva sags after pregnancy. What? You're not going to tell me yours didn't sag, now, are you? I promise I'll keep your secret.

Your First Time

Every girl remembers her great firsts. Her first kiss. Her first time making love. Her first bite of raw cookie dough. And now you can add to the list the first time you breastfeed your child. Sometimes this memorable event occurs immediately after delivery. Other times it happens after the baby has been cleaned, examined, and has been dressed in a cute hat to hide his cone-shaped head, so you won't think you gave birth to an old *Saturday Night Live* character.

But no matter when it happens, your first feeding is sure to be as exciting as any *Desperate Housewives* season finale ever was. Although you've never actually nursed before, you're filled with optimism. You've seen those ladies in coffee houses nursing their babies, chatting on their cell phones, and buttering their rolls all at the same time. How hard can it be? But then your Kodak moment doesn't go as smoothly as you had hoped when your kid can't seem to find your nipple. Or perhaps he does find it, only to suck on it for a moment before suddenly stopping. Or maybe he licks it like a Tootsie Pop and gets frustrated when he can't get to the chewy center.

If your baby doesn't start sucking madly at your breast like a prisoner during a conjugal visit, *do not worry*! These are all perfectly normal behaviors when you put your babe to your breast for the very first time. Remember, your kid didn't read those baby books like you did. He has to learn how to nurse. Like anything else, practice does indeed make perfect, and it can take several attempts before both you and your cone-headed partner get into the groove.

During this learning period, it's important to seek help from a qualified lactation specialist. This specialist can guide you through the process step by step and give you the direction and confidence you need to get through this potentially trying time. These specialists can make all the difference between loathing breastfeeding and loving it. Most hospital maternity wards have lactation specialists on staff. (In addition, breastfeeding educators, maternity nurses, and childbirth educators are all trained to provide relevant information.) If there isn't a qualified expert on hand, you can turn to a close family member or dear friend, but only if she's nursed in the past decade. Memories fade, and rules change. You don't need your Aunt Mildred telling you to put brandy on your nipple like she did for all of her kids. Sure, it may explain why your cousins like to lick the ends of batteries, but it's not sound advice. If there are no lactation experts or family members around, then get yourself out of that rice paddy and into a reputable birth center, where you can seek some help!

Hold On to What You've Got

As you travel through life, you'll find that different adventures entail getting into different positions. Yoga has its downward dog, ballet has its pas de deux, and sex has its man-I-didn't-think-my-body-would-contort-in-that-manner. Breastfeeding is no exception. In fact, there are very distinct and different positions that you can choose from in order to breastfeed your bundle of joy. You may find some more comfortable than others, especially if you had an episiotomy or a C-section. Others may be easier if you have multiple births. Either way, feel free to mix things up a bit to keep it interesting.

The Cradle Hold

You could call this the missionary position of nursing as it's the most popular of them all. It's simple and natural and, heck, you conquered it at the age of three, when you held your baby dolls. This is a one-size-fits-all hold. If you can sit up (which is no easy feat for a woman who just passed a kid through her groin), then you should be able to do it. Simply hold your baby in your arms, with his head in the crook of your elbow, and tilt your baby's body so that his belly touches yours. If your baby's body is facing up, your breast would have to make an almost impossible turn to hit its target (not unlike the bullet that killed President Kennedy, if the conspiracy theory holds true). Once his belly and yours make contact, you're good to go.

The Lying-Down Hold

Otherwise known as the lazy lima bean hold, this position is used to feed your baby while you're lying down. It's a great position if your delivery has left you with stitches or if you're feeding late at night and want to watch Letterman's top-ten list. Just lie down on one side and have your baby lie down next to you, again with his body facing yours. Support your breast with one hand and cradle your baby in the crook of your elbow to raise him to your breast if necessary. You can use pillows under your head, back, or legs, but don't put any under your baby since they pose a suffocation risk to newborns. Chances are you have plenty of spare pillows lying around as they offered more support than your husband did during your pregnancy.

The Football Hold

The football hold was given its name because it resembles the way a football player holds onto a football. Personally I hate the name because I hate all things football. I never did before I had a kid, but now my husband uses football as an excuse to get out of baby duty. "Can't miss the big game, hon!" "I'll be there as soon as they score." And since football time is like dog years, one minute on the clock takes seven minutes in real time. I wonder if my husband would be equally as accepting if I sat on my ass all weekend watching re-runs of *Beverly Hills, 90210*. But I digress.

To attain this stupidest-game-in-the-Universe hold, simply sit up in bed or in a comfy chair with your arm by your side and place a pillow underneath your forearm. Next, place your baby on top of your arm so that his head is in your hand, his back is supported by your forearm, and his legs are tucked under your armpit. In this case, make sure that his body is facing up. Because you have two arms and two breasts, this is the perfect position in which to nurse twins.

The Choke Hold

This one is not intended for nursing. Rather, this is the position you dream of giving your mother-in-law, your nosy neighbor, or anyone else who offers you unsolicited advice about breastfeeding. You've no doubt dealt with these people during your pregnancy when they freely shared their advice and horror stories. Unfortunately, they don't go away now that your placenta is gone; in fact, they tend to stick around until your kid is grown. They're constantly hovering nearby to voice their opinions on your discipline techniques, how selfish you are if you decide to only have one child, and how your new hairstyle really doesn't complement your face (they're an all-around annoyance.)

Just like the downward dog and the pas-de-deux, these nursing positions will feel awkward the first time you try them. But keep at it. Experiment with the different holds and don't give up. After time, you'll feel so comfortable holding your baby and nursing, you'll be able to nurse *and* cook dinner *and* pay some bills all at the same time. After all, we women are as good at multitasking as we are at faking orgasms—and we all know how good we are at that.

Latch On, Latch Off

If you learn only one thing from this book, it's the importance of getting your kid to latch onto your breast correctly. If he doesn't latch on correctly, he may not be able to get the milk that he so desperately needs. Also, a bad latch leads to sore nipples, which leads to pain, which leads to Similac.

The first thing to do to get a good latch is make sure that your baby's mouth lines up with your nipple properly. For this, you'll need a multitude of pillows, folded receiving blankets, and hydraulic lifts—anything to raise your baby into proper alignment. (For a visual image, imagine you're aiming your nipple for the roof of his mouth.) Then, and this is *vital*, make sure that your baby opens his mouth wide before latching on so that it engulfs as much of your areola as possible. Since the milk is stored behind the areola, your kid won't be able suck the milk out if he's only attached to your nipple. (Don't worry if he can't take in your *entire* areola since pregnancy may have caused it to grow as large as a York Peppermint Pattie.) After his mouth is latched onto your areola, the milk can flow as freely as boxed wine at a redneck convention.

In order to get your baby's mouth in place, it's crucial that he open his mouth as wide as possible. Mother Nature helps this process along by giving your kid the "rooting instinct." When stimulated, this rooting instinct makes him turn his head toward your breast and open his mouth wide. I'm not sure why it's given the name *rooting,* but I'll just file that with other parental things I'll never understand, like why we bundle up our kids like Eskimos when it's 80 degrees outside, and why we keep track of their ages in such a neurotic manner (Little Johnny just turned nineteen-and-three-quarter months old today).

To stimulate this rooting instinct, hold your breast with your thumb above your areola and your fingers supporting it underneath. Then tickle your little tyke's lower lip with your nipple until his mouth is wide open. Wait for it . . . wait for it . . . then, BAM! The instant he looks like he's about to bite into a Big Mac, quickly bring his head into your breast so that his mouth engulfs as much of your areola as possible. And I do mean quickly. There's only a second when his mouth is open wide enough to fit properly, so shove him on fast! You don't have to worry about hurting him since your breasts are made of pillowy-soft tissue. If they were made out of brick veneer, this would not be the best way to go.

If you're having trouble getting your baby's mouth to open wide enough, try opening yours, too. Even newborns are able to imitate facial movements. In fact, you're probably already opening your mouth when trying to get your kid to latch. That's because Mother Nature gave you a "show your baby how to instigate his root-ing instinct" instinct. If, after all your attempts, he still doesn't open his mouth wide enough, take the index finger of the hand that's holding your breast, put it in that gully right above his chin, and nudge it down. What you shouldn't do, however, is squeeze his cheeks together. This will overload the rooting instinct, confuse him as to which way to turn his head, and create baby gridlock.

Once you get your baby latched on, check out the placement of his tongue. His tongue should be located underneath your breast, thus creating a strong suction that rivals any toilet-bowl plunger. Then look at his lips. They should be pursed and curled over, not tucked underneath. In other words, they should look like a fish mouth.

If your kid didn't take in much of your areola, his tongue isn't below your breast, he doesn't have fish mouth, or you're experience pain (not discomfort, but pain), *stop nursing immediately*. Nursing with a bad latch will only irritate your nipples and make nursing hurt. To unlatch, take your nipple out of his mouth. But don't pull it out! This will turn your nipple into a worn-out chew toy in no time. Instead, simply put your finger between his mouth and your breast to break the suction and pop him off you like a cork.

Yes, I know that this will all seem overwhelming at first as you try to hold his head, grasp your breast, aim your nipple, and open his mouth. It's sort of like playing lactation Twister with your body tied up in a knot. That's why it's a good idea to get help from a lactation specialist when you're first learning. It's also a good idea to get help from your husband. Not because he knows how to achieve a proper latch, but because he can hold onto your various body parts until you can master holding them all by yourself. Believe me, your husband will be thrilled at the proposition. When your milk comes in, your breasts may be so tender you can't even hug the guy. He knows that this may be the only action he'll get for quite a while.

Breast Milk, Come on Down!

"Let down." In recent years, you've only used this term to describe how you felt when your husband forgot your anniversary. But ever since you pushed out your little papoose, this phrase has taken on a whole new meaning. Let down is now the term you use to explain how your breast milk travels from your breast tissue, through the ducts, and into the storage area behind your areola.

Let down occurs when your baby starts sucking away on your breast. This sucking action causes your body to release the hormone oxytocin, which in turn causes your milk to flow. Sounds simple, right? Wrong. Like most things that have to do with breastfeeding, things are much easier read than done. That's because your body's ability to cause let down is directly tied into your emotions. If you're feeling stressed out and overwhelmed (and what new mom isn't), the milk may be like a shy contestant on *The Price Is Right* who just won't "come on down."

If you're having trouble getting your milk to let down, take a few deep breaths and relax. Try putting a warm washcloth on your breast or give yourself a gentle breast massage. If that doesn't help, have your partner suckle your breast. Yes, I know it sounds odd to breastfeed your man, and it may even conjure up disturbing visuals during sex, but he has to push down some images he witnessed when you gave birth, so let's just call it even.

> "In the beginning, I had a hard time getting my milk to come down. I'd have to sit in a dark room, put on soft music and massage my breast. I felt like I was having an affair with myself whenever it was time to nurse."
>
> —Amy

After you get used to it, your breasts won't be stubborn about letting go of their milk, and let down will become easy. Too easy, in fact. Soon, your milk will come down when you hear your baby cry. Then it'll happen when you hear *any* baby cry. It'll come down during sex, when you're talking to the paper boy, and when you're giving an office presentation. Let down will come at the worst, most embarrassing moments, and that milk will come down in buckets. If you feel the distinct tingle of let down at a time when you don't want your milk to come down, cross your arms and push in on your nipples with the heels of your hand. This may help stop the flow quickly. If these embarrassing moments happen often, or if you just want to be safe, wear breast pads. They're like little maxi-pads for your nipples, and, like the maxi-pads, can stop a lot of embarrassing moments.

How Long Can This Keep Going On?

Your baby is latched on well, your milk is flowing as freely as Denise Richards's hair, and you can hear your baby gulping down mouthfuls of warm milk. You finally experience the amazing sensation that breastfeeding can bring. You feel calm, content, and fulfilled. But when after forty minutes of this fulfillment there's still no end in sight, your bliss turns to boredom, and you start to wonder, "How long do I have to keep this thing on me?"

When it comes to giving you an exact time how long each nursing session should last, I can't do it. Not because I don't want to. Heck, you shelled out good money to buy this book, and you should get more out of it than just something to balance a wobbly table. The reason I can't give you a specific time is because there is no exact figure. Depending on the time of day, the amount of milk that's produced, and the sucking action of your little one, it can vary more than co-hosts on *The View.*

In the early days of nursing, your body is in flux. It's tired, hormonal, and putting all its energy into producing milk. Your baby is in flux as well. He's just been through the huge ordeal of labor, although if you didn't have an epidural, his wasn't worth squat compared to yours. During these tender young days of nursing, your baby may not stay on each breast for more than a few minutes. Or he may fall asleep after only nursing on one side. On the other hand, he may suck on your breasts more than your husband did your entire honeymoon. And that's fine, too. Don't panic and think that his lack of interest or even his extreme eagerness means that something is wrong. Both you and your new life partner will figure out your own path.

In a few days, after your milk comes in, your baby will start taking more interest in nursing. The timing couldn't be more perfect since the more he drinks, the stronger your milk supply will become. Once in full swing, you should strive for at least eight feedings of *about* fifteen minutes per side (more or less, depending on how fast your baby eats and how much milk you produce) in a twenty-four hour period.

If your baby doesn't have eight feedings, you may want to pump to build up your supply. Not only will this produce more milk, but it'll also produce more bottles to be stockpiled in your freezer (your new goal in life). These bottles will soon mean more to you than your engagement ring since your husband can't use the old, "Gee, I really wish I could help with all those middle-of-the-night feedings but I can't lactate" excuse!

Keep in mind that a pump can never empty the breast the way your kid can, so it's still important to nurse as often as possible. In fact, pumps

may actually reduce your milk supply because
your breasts are never completely empty, so use
them sparingly during the first few weeks as the
supply/demand schedule is established.

In terms of when it's time to change sides,
let your baby decide. Some are delicate eaters
and take longer to finish the milk in one breast,
while others wolf it down like a chili dog at a
tailgate party. Don't be eager to take your baby
off your breast until he's done with it. At the end
of each breast's milk supply is something called
hindmilk, which is thicker and creamier than the
regular stuff. Since hindmilk has a higher fat content, it'll stick to his ribs more and allow him
to go longer between feedings (your second new
goal in life).

You may find that your baby wants to nurse
almost non-stop in the late afternoon and early
evening. This "cluster feeding" goes hand and in
hand with your baby's fussy time, when, for some
unexplained reason, your quiet kid turns into
a cranky monster who can only be consoled by
being allowed to dangle from your chest like a
nipple ring (again, very normal behavior).

Finally, when you're done feeding on one side,
don't forget to burp your kid. But don't expect
it to sound like it would if he had downed that

chili dog. A breastfed baby swallows far less air than one who's bottlefed and may not even burp at all. So don't continue to pound on your poor kid's back like a dirty rug in order to squeeze out a belch. Just a minute or so of gentle taps should suffice.

Double the Trouble

As if breastfeeding isn't hard enough to deal with if you have one kid, you had to go off and have two or more! With the help of in vitro fertilization, or just plain good luck, you are now one of the abundance of parents of multiple births! Just think of all those delicious hugs and sticky fingerprints! A couple of years from now, having two or more kids the same age will pay off big time. Your children will always have a playmate nearby, and they can help each other with the homework problems that you can't seem to figure out. But for now, while they're still helpless and young, having multiple kids means multiple problems, especially when it comes to breastfeeding.

In the fantasy world of breastfeeding twins, both babies would be hungry at the same time. They'd nurse for the same duration, one on each boob, and after a hearty meal would instantly fall asleep and stay that way throughout the night. As they grew, they'd never fight except about which deserving charity to donate their lemonade stand money to. As adults, they'd shower you with oodles of grandchildren and call you every day just to tell you how much they love you. But until all that happens, let's just get 'em fed!

Rarely does it happen that different kids will eat in the same manner. Chances are that each will have a different appetite, a different eating style, and a need for different amounts of feeding per day. This translates into feeding your babies around the clock and going out of your mind dealing with their eating idiosyncrasies. The best way to get your litter on the same schedule is to remember that crying doesn't necessarily mean that a baby is hungry. If you can satisfy them with cuddles instead of chow, you may be able to get all your babies on the same feeding schedule and relieve a lot of your stress.

Another good stress reliever is a product called the EZ2 Nurse. It's the crème de la crème of nursing pillows and specifically made for multiples. It totally surrounds your body and had deep sides that are angled inward so your kidlettes fall right into place like little Rockettes.

Above all, do everything you can to simplify your life. If you're going to pump, get a double pump so that you can express from both breasts at the same time and cut your pumping time in half. When people visit, insist they bring a stuffed turkey in lieu of a stuffed animal so that you don't have to cook. And forget about the small things for a while, like giving your babies a daily bath. It's not like they're doing anything to work up a sweat. Until life settles down, spot clean their mishaps and call it a day.

Like anything else, practice makes perfect. Experiment with different feeding positions and different products. Most of all, get lots of help. Expect frustrations and expect the unexpected. And focus on the positives, like your beautiful babies, and the fact that you can eat an additional 500 calories per kid to produce all that milk!

Side Order

There are a lot of things to keep track of after you deliver your baby. What you need to remember is which visitors are coming over which days, what gifts you've already written thank-you cards for, and if you remembered to take your morning shower (although the answer to that question is always a resounding "no"). On top of all those details, you're also expected to keep a running tally of which breast you started nursing with first so that you can alternate with the other one on your next feeding. Holy crap! You couldn't even remember to take your birth control pill, which is what got you into this mess in the first place. With so many daily feedings, how the heck are you going to keep track of it all?

Easy, girl, easy. Let's see if we can come up with a simple way to remember which breast you led off with during feeding time. You've no doubt heard of the tried-and-true method of keeping a safety pin attached to your bra and switching it back and forth after each feeding. Personally, I never liked this method very much. I had enough going on trying to get my baby latched on without having to struggle to unfasten a sharp projectile and keep it from falling into my baby's open mouth.

In lieu of the safety-pin method, might I suggest the following other ways that won't result in a having a razor-sharp needle land in your baby's gaping pie hole:

A small piece of cloth: Just cut a swatch out of any soft, washable fabric. Place it inside of your bra, and move it back and forth as needed. It's easier than wrangling a sharp pin, and it comes in handy when your kid spits up and you can't find any of the 5,000 burp cloths you have scattered around the house.

A strip of Velcro: Velcro is one of today's best inventions, along with hybrid cars and salad in a bag. Just attach a small strip onto one of your bra cups and move it back and forth as needed.

A breast pad: Not only will this help you remember which side you need to start nursing from, but it will sop up any leaks as well (from one side anyway). Sure, your breasts may look a bit lopsided when you're not nursing, but let's face it, right now your boobs are so big that no one will ever notice. Could you really tell if Tweedledee was a few pounds lighter than Tweedledum?

Feed Me!

It's amazing how fast time goes by when you have a baby. Every moment you're busy, either putting something into him or cleaning something that just came out of him. When it comes to the constant feedings, it seems as if you've given birth to the plant in *Little Shop of Horrors*. As soon as you pull off your baby from your boobs and tuck them back in for a quick rest, your kid is sucking his hand, rooting madly, or crying. Break time is over, girls; let's get back to work!

Sure, you knew that newborns can eat every two hours. What you may not have known is that the clock doesn't start ticking when you're *done* with nursing but rather when you *start*. Let's take a look to see how this plays out:

2:00 A.M.: Your baby cries to be fed. You look at your husband, either amazed that he can sleep though all the crying or amazed at what a poor job he's doing pretending to be asleep.

2:01 A.M.: You take your baby out of the crib and check his diaper to make sure it's not too wet or poopy. Yup, it's poopy. You change it in the dark because you don't want to turn on the lights and startle him so much that he won't fall back to sleep.

2:15 A.M.: Nursing begins.

2:45 A.M.: Nursing ends. Problem is, now your kid's wide awake and wants to play. This is not only because he can't tell the difference between night and day but also because you caved and turned on the lights after failing to clean that messy bottom in the dark.

3:15 A.M.: You finally get your baby back to sleep. You crawl back in bed, but now it's you who's wide awake. (It's hard to put yourself back to sleep every few hours.) You start to nod off but your husband snores loudly, scaring you and causing adrenaline to course through your veins.

3:45 A.M.: You finally fall asleep, no easy feat with adrenaline coursing through your veins.

4:15 A.M.: It's been two hours since you last started feeding your child, and he's ready to go again. You've had only thirty minutes of sleep. You're exhausted but you get up again to feed your kid—and to look for the power drill, with in order to carve wider nostrils in your hubby's face.

Since most babies eat about eight to twelve times a day, and some kids spend up to forty-five minutes nursing, you can understand why you need to call your mother right this instant and thank her for everything she ever did for you. You used to be so determined to nurse exclusively for a year, but now in your exhausted state, you totally get why so many mothers decide to supplement formula at nighttime or even quit nursing altogether. In fact, you're thinking your few weeks of nursing should do just fine.

Yes, nursing is hard! Very hard. In fact, some women find it the hardest maternal thing they ever had to do. Fortunately with kids, the only thing constant is change (and a steady trail of those poopy diapers). Newborns grow as fast as Sea-Monkeys, and every day they take in more milk and can last longer between feedings. Plus, they get better and better at nursing and can get the milk out in less time. This will translate into more continuous sleep, less exhaustion, and less resentment toward your spouse. That is, of course, unless he snores, in which case you'll resent him for a lifetime.

If your kid is six months old and still waking up during the night to be fed, chances are it's because of habit instead of hunger. Let him fuss in his crib a bit before you get up to see if he'll fall back to sleep. Pat him on the back to comfort him instead of offering him a midnight snack. Then go out and get yourself a good baby sleeping book (check out the resources listed in the appendix at the end of the book for suggestions) and learn all the tricks to the sleeping trade. Once your baby sleeps through the night, you can, too.

Out of Control

If you have the kind of personality that's prone to being organized and likes to be in control, giving birth will throw a wrench in your system that's larger than any found in a Craftsman tool set. If having a clean house, a washed car, and always being on time is your kind of thing, you're in for a rocky ride, my friend. Having a new baby and a well-scheduled day do not go hand in hand.

Maybe you think you should be in charge of when your baby eats and sleeps. Yes, if you knew exactly when you'd feed him and put him down for a nap, you could have far more control of your day. You could run errands, return calls, and meet girlfriends for lunch. Yup, that's what you'll do. You'll follow a rigid schedule! The only problem is that your baby won't follow it with you.

I'm sure you've heard of women who put their babies on a schedule from the moment they were born. They took consistent naps and ate at consistent times. Me, I find those stories funnier than the Apple computer commercials. I'm not saying that your baby won't have a schedule, but it won't happen until your schnookums is about three months old. It's at that time when he'll fall into a natural rhythm of eating and sleeping (and even pooping!). But for now, you just need to grin and bear it and go with the flow.

Some women (code name for "your mother-in-law") will tell you that newborns don't really need to eat all the time and yours is just being manipulative. It's like he's pissed off because you force him to sleep on his back instead of his cozy belly. But there's nothing manipulative about your baby's behavior. The truth is that a new-born's stomach is very small and can't hold much food. And denying him food just because it's not his scheduled feeding time is not the advised approach. Not only can it lead to poor weight gain in your child, but it can lead to a low milk supply in your breasts. During your baby's first few precious months outside the womb, welcome him with open arms and feed him on demand. It'll keep your baby, and your boobies, healthy.

As the weeks pass and your baby gets bigger, his stomach will, too. Then he'll be able to load up on milk as if each meal were Sunday dinner and last longer between feedings. It's at that time that a schedule will form. You'll have more control of your day, and you'll begin to get more organized. But don't jump the gun and start thinking that means you'll once again have a clean house and a tidy car and can arrive to places on time. Instead, you'll be content if you can simply find time to pee when you want to.

Wake Up Little Cutie, Wake Up

If your newborn is sleeping so well at night that you're struggling with the dilemma of whether or not to wake him for feedings, consider yourself lucky. Most new parents would give their Bugaboo strollers to have that kind of problem, so keep that information to yourself or suffer the consequence of having no friends to invite to little Junior's birthday parties.

The question of whether or not to wake up a sleeping baby is like whether or not to refrigerate peanut butter. And like the peanut butter dilemma, people have very strong and varied viewpoints. After years of study (okay, by asking a large handful of friends), I've found that people base the decision of where to put their peanut butter on where their mothers kept it. Not so with the sleeping question. For that, you have to listen to another person: your pediatrician. He should always be the voice of reason when it comes to your baby's health concerns. Whether it be during your baby's regular checkup or during those panicked calls you place when you think that your child is dying because of some oddly shaped poop, your pediatrician is your go-to guy.

Oddly enough, viewpoints about whether or not to wake a sleeping baby for feeding time will vary from pediatrician to pediatrician. Many advise you to let him sleep. Assuming that he's gaining weight at a good rate and you have a good supply of milk, your pediatrician may tell you not to worry about such things . . . or, for that matter, the shape of your kid's poop. Other pediatricians, however, may say to wake him up at certain intervals to nurse to avoid dehydration and to keep your milk supply strong.

"I was so lucky that I had a good sleeper, but I was still constantly exhausted. Just because my baby slept didn't mean I did. I was up all night worrying that she'd stop breathing or that she'd dehydrate, so I'd keep pinching her hand to see if her skin would snap back."

—Carol

If your pediatrician suggests that you wake your baby-kins for feedings, let me offer some words of wisdom. Waking up a sleeping baby and getting him to eat is harder than getting Jon Stewart to be bipartisan. You're always walking the delicate line of waking him enough to drink but not so much that he won't be able to fall right back to sleep.

Like all things in life, timing is important. If you can, avoid waking your baby when his eyelids are fluttering and his body is doing those cute twitching movements. When this happens, he's no doubt in REM sleep, otherwise known as deep sleep, and he will be harder to wake. If you wake him but he's too tired to drink, unbutton his jammies a bit so he won't be so warm and snug. Stroke the palms of his hands and soles of his feet as well. Chances are, even if you do everything right, he may still be drowsy and won't take in more food than Nicole Richie. But at least it will be some and that will be good, for even that small nosh counts for something.

After about six weeks, when your baby has put on some weight and your milk production is in high gear, your pediatrician may tell you that waking up your baby to eat isn't necessary any more (depending on other factors like weight gain, hydration, and the number of poopy and wet diapers). Then you can all sleep better and be ready for the next child-rearing challenge that comes your way.

Diaper Detail

One of the great frustrations of nursing is that your boobs aren't see-through. Unlike bottles, which come with convenient markings along the side, boobs only come with a few new stretch marks. Because of this, you have no idea how much milk your little one is actually ingesting. It's enough to drive a postpartum, hormone-riddled woman crazy, although that's not saying a whole heck of a lot since she's pretty much crazy all the time anyway.

This is an especially strange phenomenon because our bodies have become perfected following millions of years of evolution. We have fingernails to protect our sensitive fingertips, eyebrows to stop debris from falling in our eyes, and underarm hair to do whatever the hell it's supposed to do. So why can't our boobies have tiny little dip-sticks to clue us in on how much our kids are drinking?

Because of this, many women fear they're not making enough milk. Some think this is because their breasts are small. Others think it's because they may not have become engorged or haven't leaked (again, not a sign). And still more think it's true because their babies cry in the late afternoon and early evening and want to nurse for hours. But most babies get fussy during this time. It's what new moms refer to as *arsenic hour* because it coincides with the busiest part of our days, when we become so frazzled that we're tempted to just end it all.

Fortunately, there *is* a way of knowing if your baby is getting enough nourishment. True, we may not have markings on our breasts, but your baby has markings of his own, and you can see these markings inside of his diapers. During the first few days of nursing, when your baby only drinks a small amount of colostrum, don't expect much in the waste-management department.

Only a couple of wee-wees and a poop-poop or two should suffice. But after about day six, when your milk has had enough time to come in, the big diaper turnover begins. It's then that you can expect your baby-kins to have *about* six wet diapers per day, plus three mustardy yellow poop-ity poops. (Because breast milk is so easily absorbed, there may be less, or even no poopy diapers at all for a few days. Always call your pediatrician with any concerns.) After a couple of months, as your baby's digestive system matures, you should have fewer poops (although what they lack in quantity, they'll make up for in quality and can seem to be the size of your baby himself!)

You may have already been advised by your doctor and your nightstand-full of books to keep a running tally of your baby's diaper contents for the first few weeks of his life. You may also have been told to keep a log of when you breastfeed, how long your kid stays on each breast, his sleeping habits, and the combined batting average of the American League teams. Personally, I think the six remaining brain cells you have left after pregnancy have enough going on just remembering stuff like where you live, but log away if you must.

The important thing to remember is you should feel confident your baby is eating enough if he regains all of his post birth weight loss in two weeks, nurses eight to twelve times a day, swallows at the breast, and starts packing on about half a pound a week. If your baby isn't measuring up, make sure he's latched on properly and that he's getting enough feedings. Make sure that you're not exercising or dieting in excess, not taking birth control pills, and that you haven't had cosmetic work done on your breasts in the past.

If you're having any problems feeding your baby enough milk, consult a lactation specialist, who will advise you about your latch, different pumping techniques, herbs and teas, and various solutions to your specific problems. Lactation specialists can solve most lactation problems and are a nursing woman's breast friend!

Chapter 3

"Nursing" Your Wounds

I don't know how other mammals do it. They pop out their young without the help of epidurals or ice chips, and then they take to nursing without a care in the world. Their faces don't grimace. Their nipples don't crack. And I've never seen any other mammal in the entire animal kingdom wear a nipple shield to draw out an inverted teat.

But the human mammal is like no other. In fact, we seem to have nothing *but* problems when it comes to nursing our young. Unlike our other bodily functions, like burping and farting, which occur without effort, breastfeeding seems to require nothing but. And the help we need to ease our pain isn't found in nature, but rather

69

on the shelves of drugstores across the country.
I don't know of one breastfeeding mother who
lasted the duration without the help from something with a bar code.

In fact, how our foremothers survived at
all without modern day luxuries like TiVo and
Tupperware is beyond me. That's why, as much
as you might suffer from nursing problems, take
a moment to reflect on the stamina of our procre-
ating past, women who survived through early
motherhood without the benefit of painkillers,
breast pumps, and those wonderful stool soften-
ers to get them through their first postpartum
poops.

If you're a nursing mother, there's a good
chance that you'll become a victim of one or
more nursing problems. Some may be mild and
need only the help of your own breast milk, while
others may make you so miserable that you'll be
tempted to quit nursing altogether. But as frustrating as they can be, try to stick with it. In most
cases, nursing problems last only a day or two.
They usually occur during the first few weeks of
breastfeeding, when both you and your baby are
still working out the kinks in the system. After
your milk production adjusts and you and your
baby become as in sync as professional ribbon

dancers, most of your nursing problems will be behind you. But until that day, here's the low-down of some common problems that take place after let down.

Chapped Nips

Although your vagina took quite a beating during delivery, it was your nipples that went through the biggest transformation during pregnancy. Your areolas, once small and pillowy soft, may have morphed into giant, dark, disc-like saucers. Your nipples, which were once spongy and malleable, may now be so big and hard that you can use them to pry the lids off of paint cans. And now that you're nursing, the situation may get even worse.

That's because if nursing isn't done correctly, it can cause this delicate part of your anatomy to become irritated and often cracked. Sometimes this cracking even draws blood, which in turn, leads to scabs. Once this happens, the pain you must endure to nurse can often be excruciating. If pain is Mother Nature's way of telling you that something's wrong, then your nipples are screaming at you like Sam Kinison.

Although all nipples are fair game for soreness, the nipples of women whose skin is fair or delicate are especially vulnerable to the abuse of a kid's sucking action. Also, if your child is a voracious eater, he can wind up chewing your nipples like a cheap cut of meat. But even dark-skinned women with babies who eat so delicately they extend their pinkies when they indulge can still experience the pain of sore nipples.

Far and above the most common reason for getting sore nipples is a bad latch. At the very beginning of your breastfeeding endeavor, when nursing doesn't come as naturally as breathing or applying mascara while you drive, it's vital that you check your baby's latch each and every time you nurse. Make sure that his mouth is open wide before you put him on your breast, and make visually sure that he's taken in most, if not all, of your areola. If he's not, pull that sucker off you like a chigger before he can do any damage.

But I'll be honest here. Even if your kid latches on like chrome to a bumper, you may still experience some discomfort. Let's face it. Every time your baby nurses, he's essentially giving a hickey to one of the most sensitive parts of your body. Then, once he's done, your raw and moist nipples are exposed to irritation when they're put back

in their bra. How could there *not* be any damage
with that kind of abuse? It'd be like running a
power sander over your tongue every two hours
around the clock.

Here are a few things to do to prevent sore
nipples and ease the pain if it occurs:

- **Air out your nipples before you put
  them back in your bra.** Pull down the
  front flaps of your nursing bra and let them
  run wild. You'll still get the support you
  need, and the air will dry them off to prevent chafing.

- **To heal cracks, apply some breast milk
  to your nipples and your entire areola
  after each feeding.** If you'd like, you can
  also use a topical cream like medical-grade
  lanolin or A&D ointment. Remember that
  not all creams are created equal and, since
  your baby will be ingesting some with
  every feeding, the cream needs to be pure.
  Don't use petroleum jelly, alcohol, soaps,
  or moisturizing lotions or anything that
  contains chemicals.

- **If your nipples are very irritated and
  sore, cover them in a breast shell when
  they're not in use.** A breast shell is a

plastic protective cage-like device that looks like you're putting your nipples in a *Silence of the Lambs* Halloween costume.

- **Try a salt-water bath.** To ease the pain, dip your nipples in a coffee mug full of warm, salty water (add about a tablespoon of salt to each mug).
- **Give your breasts some tea—a tea bag, that is.** Soak tea bags in cold water and apply them to the sore area.

Sore nipples, and the effects they can cause, are not pleasant to deal with. I realize how unnerving it is to take your baby off your breast and see your blood on his mouth—or worse still, to realize that the scab that was there before you nursed is now nowhere in sight. But I promise that your baby will not get sick from either of these scenarios. You, however, may experience nausea, dry heaves, and a bad case of the heeby-jeebies just thinking about it.

The best thing you can do to help sore nipples is give the situation time. Your body has had to get used to a lot of painful things in the past, like braces, acne, and unattractive cropped pants. It will get used to this, too. In the meantime, pamper your nipples. Slather on the breast milk, keep them dry, and give them some tea. I know it can be sad to look at your nipples and remember how lovely they were before breastfeeding. But if you take a hand mirror and check out what delivery did to your vagina, your nipples won't look so bad by comparison.

Flat or Inverted Nipples

Our nipples are like little accordions that can grow larger or smaller, depending on whether there's a cold breeze or a hot hunk around. But no matter how cold or "hot" they get, some nipples stay flat or even recess. If you are the owner of nipples with erectile dysfunction, you may worry that having flat or inverted nipples may cause more nursing problems. Take a deep breath and relax. The truth is that when you nurse, your baby doesn't actually suck from your nipple anyway. Instead, he latches on to your areola since that's where your milk is stored. Then the milk squirts out through the holes in the nipples. So you see, the pop-up quality to nipples is purely for decoration.

If your nipples are vertically challenged, make sure you teach proper latching techniques to your newborn right from the get-go. Before your milk comes in, your areolas will be their softest and most supple, so it's much easier for your baby to grasp hold of them. Once it comes in, your breasts will be like hard watermelons, making the latch-on more difficult. Because of this, make sure that you consult a lactation specialist in the hospital and nurse often to get the most practice time.

If you have flat or inverted nipples, there are things you can do to try to get them to come out of hiding. The Internet is filled with ads for penile enhancement products, so it's only fair there are products to make your nipples stand up at attention as well. The first line of defense are breast shells, plastic cup-like contraptions that you wear on your nipples to squeeze them out like toothpaste from a tube. A breast pump is another good way to draw out your nipples before a feeding. You can also try to elongate your nipple manually. Gently grasp your breast in your hand, with your thumb on top and your fingers underneath, and push your hand inward toward your chest.

You should avoid using pacifiers and bottles since it may be confusing for your baby to go from a shorter nipple to one that's long and hard (insert your own sex joke here, since mine will inevitably be edited out). In fact, you may want to completely omit them for four to six weeks until your baby is able to nurse like a pro. (There is conflicting evidence on when and whether it's good to use pacifiers. Pacifier use has been associated with a decrease in SIDS. If you're concerned, you may not want to use the pacifier during the four- to six-week period, then strike a healthy balance between how often and when you provide it.)

But by far the best thing you can do if you have flat or inverted nipples is to see a lactation specialist (ideally before you give birth, and if not immediately afterward). Don't wait until your baby is born and you're in such extreme pain that you don't nurse very often, leaving you so engorged you think your breasts will rip in two. A lactation specialist will give you hands-on instruction about your nipples and your latch and will help solve all of your breastfeeding woes. If you had problems nursing in the past due to inverted nipples and are planning for another baby, there's a simple medical procedure that can be done in the doctor's office to correct the problem.

As you can see, flat or inverted nipples do not mean "no" to nursing. There are plenty of ways to charm a nipple out of its hole. Just stick with it, see a lactation specialist, and don't let your low nipples get you down.

Bowling Balls for Breasts

A few days after your baby is born, your milk will come in, and you'll no doubt become engorged. This may continue the first few weeks of nursing, while you and your baby try to get in the groove. During this time, your breasts will feel hot, tender, and very sore when they're full. This will likely be especially true in the morning, when you have the most milk. In fact, it's very common to lift yourself off the bed and see two wet marks staring up at you where your breasts have just been.

With breastfeeding, the most common flaw in the system is that you're not always there with the goods when it's feeding time. Oftentimes you're stuck in a long line at the bank, or in bumper-to-bumper traffic. Sometimes your baby is asleep when your milk comes in and seems to take the longest nap of his short life. When this happens, your breasts become full with milk and are sore and leaky.

You bear through the pain until you can get to your baby and then throw him on your chest like a beautiful brooch. You expect relief, but all you get are tears when your baby can't get his mouth around your overblown hooters. It's like trying to latch on to a big balloon . . . and I'm taking the giant kind that floats down Fifth Avenue during the Thanksgiving Day parade. Now you're in pain, your baby is in tears, and your leaky breasts are causing the room to fill up like the *Titanic.*

So what's an engorged mother to do? The most important thing to do is to stop the engorgement before it starts. Stick to regular feeding times as much as possible. Arrange errands so that you're able to be with your baby at regular intervals. If your boobs are filling up and your kid isn't interested in eating, pump a bit to keep yourself comfortable. If you're so engorged that he can't get his mouth around your areola, pump to relieve the pressure and soften things up. If you don't have a pump, give yourself a "hand job" and express some of the milk yourself. (To learn how to express by hand, see the resources listed in the appendix at the back of the book.) You can also take a warm shower to allow some milk to leak until your breasts are soft enough to allow your baby to latch.

To relieve the pain of engorgement, toss a couple of bags of frozen peas on your breasts. Another trick is to peel off the outer leaves of a chilled green cabbage (not the purple kind, which stains), crush or break them, and put them inside your bra. Green cabbage contains a chemical that helps relieve the pain of engorgement, and crushing the leaves helps release it for absorption by your skin. Just be sure you keep the cabbage in there for no longer than two hours at a time; any longer than that, and it will reduce milk production. Be prepared: Because leaking will occur, it's a good idea to use breast pads, tissues, or paper towels to soak up your excess milk. It also helps to wear one of your looser bras. The looser the bra, the less constricting it will be and the better you'll feel. Tight bras will reduce milk production, as well.

To help reduce leaking, press the heels of your hands into your nipples. You can press your forearms against your breasts as well. Anything that applies pressure to the breast and pushes the areola into the chest will stop the flow of milk. And never be without a sweater or long-sleeved shirt in public so you can tie it around your shoulders (in a flashback to the preppy look of the 1980s) to conceal any wet spots.

The worst of your engorgement problems will happen after your milk first comes in. Then the problems will occur only if you miss a feeding or begin to wean. After a few weeks, engorgement won't be as much of a problem as your body adjusts to your schedule. Until then, keep peas in the freezer, a cabbage in your fridge, and a sweater in your diaper bag, and avoid running errands around feeding time. In fact, why not just avoid running errands altogether and have your husband do them instead? Up till now he's been spared the pains of motherhood, from morning sickness to the episiotomy. The least he can do is pick up the dry cleaning.

A Nasty Clog

Everything is going great. Your baby's nursing well, and you're confident you have a handle on the whole ordeal. Then almost overnight, you find a painful lump in your breast. Unfortunately, it seems you have the common aliment knows as a breast clog. Fortunately, your baby is the answer to your pain because he has the strength to suck out even the most stubborn clog!

"When I had a clog I was in so much pain,
I had my husband help me suck it out. It was
then I realized one of the secret reasons why it's easier
to raise a child in a two-parent household.

—Anonymous mom

Treating Clogs

If you have a clog, there are certain ways you can nurse to best harness your baby's powers. First, make sure you begin nursing on the clogged side first. That's when your baby is the hungriest and offers the most suck for the buck. When placing him on your breast, you must also aim his chin toward to the clog since the lower mouth has the most sucking power.

If the clog is stubborn or very painful, you can ready it for draining by applying heat before you nurse. If you're one of those amazing moms who can actually find time in her busy day to take a shower, run the warm water over the clogged breast for several minutes. For the rest of you, that is, those who can barely find time to inhale, simply place a warm washcloth over the affected area. Once it is warmed, massage the clog by gently pushing it toward your nipple. (Don't rub it in circles.)

If you have a clog in your breast, give your nipple the old look-see to check for a small white blister. If there is one (*gross!*), it's no doubt the cause of the problem and will need to be popped (*double gross!*). To do this, soak your nipple in warm water for ten minutes either in a bath, a warm basin of water, or even a coffee mug, and then, with a sterile needle, pop open the blister. Yes, it's disgusting and will make you want to start feeding your kid Power Bars from now on, but it's all part and parcel of the process.

Preventing Clogs

If you find that your breasts clog as easily as a toilet at Shea Stadium, it might behoove you to take lecithin. A 1,200 mg tablet, three times a day, may actually prevent clogs, but check with your doctor first. I'm sure he'll okay it, but I have say these things for legal reasons since I'm sure there'll be one reader who will take lecithin, get a hangnail, and come after me.

To avoid breast clogs, keep engorgement to a minimum and change nursing positions frequently. Breast milk is like a shark: It has to keep in constant motion. If you allow it to stew in its own juices too long, it tends to thicken up like gravy and cause a clog. Most importantly, once a clog forms, *do not stop nursing!* This will only make matters worse and can lead to far worse things than a simple clog.

So if almost overnight you find a painful mass in your breast, relax. All you need are the Drano sucking powers of your little one's jaws. And you thought having a kid around wouldn't be helpful until he was old enough to start taking out the garbage!

Mastitis

Getting mastitis is every mother's worst nightmare. It's right up there with dropping your kid on the hardwood floor or losing him at the mall because you played hide-and-seek, got distracted by a pair of cute summer slingbacks, and forgot to actually "seek." If you thought a breast clog was bad, it's nothing compared to mastitis, a far more serious and longer-lasting condition. Mastitis can make you feel even sicker than you felt the time you thought Long Island iced tea was simply tea made in Long Island.

When you come down with mastitis, your breasts become incredibly achy and tender. Even a strong gust of wind can bring you to tears. You'll have a high fever of 101 or more, and feel very, very, very, tired . . . even more so than your regular very, very tired. In fact, your whole body will feel like it's been run over by a truck. And I'm talking a Mack truck, not one of those wimpy ass pickups that you borrow from a friend when you have an appliance to move.

Sometimes mastitis is caused by a breast clog that wasn't nursed often enough to drain. Other times, it's brought on because you didn't alternate the breast you started with during each feeding. Still other times it's caused by a germ that gets passed from your baby's mouth, through your cracked nipple, and into your milk ducts. Once there, the germ sets up shop and goes forth and multiplies . . . exponentially. That's why almost overnight you can go from feeling healthy to feeling heinous.

> "I'm never sick. I was even up and around when
>
> I had a concussion. But I stayed in bed for days
>
> when I got mastitis and wanted to die."
>
> —Lizzy

If you start to feel achy and tired and have painful breasts and a high fever, call your doctor right away. With treatment (usually a round of antibiotics), your breasts will be up and around in no time. Until then, to relieve the pain, apply cold packs and take Tylenol. Also, even though you'd rather stick needles in your eye, keep on nursing! I know that every milk duct in your being is pleading with you to start weaning, but that would be the very worst thing you could do right now. If you don't keep draining your milk supply, the infection can get worse and lead to an abscess, a condition that will make mastitis seem like a mosquito bite. If pus appears at the nipple, you must see a doctor to have the abscess drained right away. Oh, and finally, like the books suggest, be sure to get plenty of rest. (Yeah, like that's gonna happen when you have a new baby. Some of those books are a funnier read than *The Devil Wears Prada*.)

You're Abscessed!

When it comes to breastfeeding ailments, there's one that towers over all the rest. It's the Super Bowl of soreness. The pinnacle of pain.

We're talking about . . . the breast abscess! The biggest scare to hit your breasts since silicone implants! Not only is the breast abscess the most severe, it will mark the end of the world as you know it. You'll feel so miserable that you'll long for the old days of motherhood when you spent your days in total exhaustion cleaning up projectile poops.

A breast abscess is an infection deep inside your breast that causes a painful buildup of pus. But the symptoms go much further than just having a red, swollen, painful mass. A breast abscess also causes you to suffer from headache, fatigue, fever, nausea, and vomiting. Still, no matter how much pain you're in, no matter how close to death's door you feel, you will still have to wake up around the clock to nurse your young! And you wonder why they ever came up with Mother's Day!

The most common way to get a breast abscess is to stop or limit nursing when you have a clogged duct or mastitis. As we've discussed, that's a big nursing no-no because it can only make matters worse. It's like throwing fuel on a fire or telling your husband he doesn't do enough around the house right after a big argument about money.

If you have an abscess, see your doctor right away. Do not pass *go*, or even that yummy doughnut shop on the way that makes those fantastic fritters. Once there, you'll be given an ultrasound to locate the mass. But unlike the ultrasounds you had during pregnancy, this one won't reveal any fingers, toes, or an enormous penis that will make your husband proud until he's told it's merely the umbilical chord. Instead, this ultrasound will show only a big mass of pus that will have to be surgically drained. After the procedure, you'll be prescribed a full round of antibiotics, instructed to drink lots of fluids, and again, told to get a lot of bed rest. Not easy when you have a newborn who requires more attention than Paris Hilton.

If the mass is severe or in a bad location, you'll be asked to nurse only with the healthy breast. The infected breast will then need to be pumped and dumped and the milk thrown out like last year's fashions. After a few days, when the antibiotics kick in, you'll feel like a person again. You'll have a whole new outlook on life and appreciate the little things like morning dew, a good parking spot, and of course, those fantastic fritters.

Soothe the Savage Yeast

Man oh man, why is yeast such a problem for
us women? It's as if God punished Eve for giving Adam the apple by stuffing a loaf of Wonder
Bread up her crotch. Since then, yeast has caused
our vaginas to itch and burn and generally make
our lives miserable.

But our vaginas aren't the only body part
that can get affected by yeast. It can make our
nipples pretty miserable as well. At least it can
while we breastfeed. That's because yeast thrives
in moist, dark, and warm environments, and putting wet nipples in thick nursing bras is like giving them a beachfront cottage in the Hamptons.
The yeast will be so comfortable that it'll unpack
its bags, stock the fridge with goodies, and party
on down.

The signs of yeast (also known as thrush or
candida) aren't as obvious as a breast clog or mastitis. But the symptoms are fairly typical. For one,
your nipples become incredibly sore. They will
burn and itch, appearing red and even blistery.
But unlike the immediate pain that's caused by
an incorrect latch, the pain of yeast usually occurs
at the end of nursing. Yeast that affects the nipple

can also affect your baby's tongue! After nursing, his tongue may be coated with a white substance that's denser than your breast milk. Your little one might also have white dots inside his mouth and on his tongue. Another sign of yeast is that your baby gets a bad diaper rash and his diapers emit the odor of freshly baked bread!

A yeast infection can come on for no apparent reason, and you don't need to have a vaginal yeast infection to get it on your nipples. Although there is no rhyme or reason to getting this type of infection, there is one common way to bring it on: taking a round of antibiotics. Antibiotics are equal opportunity destroyers that kill both the good and the bad bacteria in your system. That's why, when you're taking antibiotics, yeast can grow more than the kudzu vine of the South.

If you suspect a yeast infection, call your doctor right away to get a prescription for an antifungal cream to put on your nipples. You'll also be advised to eat plenty of yogurt with live cultures in order to build up the good bacteria in your system and discourage the yeast. If you don't like yogurt, you can take acidophilus pills instead. Your baby may be treated as well, even if he doesn't have a white film on his tongue or a diaper that brings back fond memories of Grandma's buttermilk biscuits.

Like most all other nursing problems, an ounce of prevention is worth a pound of pain. So do yourself a favor and follow these simple tips:

- **If you're ever on antibiotics, eat plenty of yogurt.** Follow this advice whether you're breastfeeding or not, and make sure the yogurt you choose contains live cultures. You can also take acidophilus pills.
- **After nursing, air-dry your nipples before putting them back in the barn.**
- **Change your nursing pads often.** This way, you're not keeping damp material close to your nipples. Remember, moisture equals misery!
- **Wash and dry your breast pump.** Do the same for all pacifiers, breast shells, bottle nipples, and anything else that comes in contact with your baby's mouth or your breast.
- **Use 100 percent cotton material for your bras and breast pads.** Be sure to clean them in hot water and dry them thoroughly before putting them on.

- **Expose your hooters to sunlight.** Yeast thrives in the dark, so give your boobs some fun in the sun for a few minutes every day.
- **If you have a yeast infection, keep your husband's mouth away from your nipples.** Yeast is contagious and can cause him to suffer from athlete's foot or jock itch. (Although if you still resent him for not being able to lactate, you can just keep this fact to yourself.)

As is true of most other nursing problems, breastfeeding with a yeast infection can be painful. In this case, it can actually be excruciating. But that doesn't give you license to stop. As you know, ladies, if you don't drain your tank, it can make your milk stank!

Too Much of a Good Thing

Because it's impossible to visually tell how much milk your baby is drinking, most women worry that their bodies aren't producing enough. But some women don't have that worry. That's because their bodies produce more milk than a dairy farm. At first, you'd think that producing too much wouldn't be much of a problem, but there are definite challenges and pains that can happen when your bra cup runneth over.

To begin with, breasts that are very full of milk are more prone to engorgement, breast clogs, and mastitis. Your baby can't possibly consume all the milk you produce, so it stays in your ducts and causes more problems than teens on spring break. In addition, let down can be incredibly painful since the milk comes down in full force.

When too much breast milk is produced, mommies aren't the only ones who suffer. Their babies tend to suffer right along with them. They often gag when they eat, as they can't swallow fast enough, and latching on can be a challenge since the milk squirts all over them like a shower. Babies who have an overabundance of milk at their disposal can have various weight issues as well. Either they drink more than they should because it's so readily available, or they push away at the breast in frustration and don't get enough. Also, the makeup of the breast milk itself can pose problems. Since there's so much milk, the babies ingest more foremilk and are full by the time they get to the thicker hindmilk.

Since foremilk tends to be higher in lactose, these babies can have tummy problems. Plus, because they don't get enough hindmilk, they tend to be hungry an hour later, as if they just downed a breast full of Chinese food.

If you have a gallon of milk in your pint-sized containers, here are a few things you can do to help minimize the problems:

Don't switch your newborn to the second breast until you're sure that he's emptied the first one. That way he should get enough hind-milk to satisfy him for a few hours between feedings. If necessary, only feed him from one breast. If the other breast is uncomfortably full, express just enough to be comfortable. Don't empty it all, or your body will think that your baby actually needs that much milk and will continue to produce it. Start with the fuller breast on your next feeding.

Forget the all-cotton reusable breast pads. They're not strong enough to absorb your hefty leaks. Instead, go for the heavy-duty disposable pads with the plastic liners. They'll do a much better job of preventing leaks so that your clothes don't have that tie-dye effect on the nipple area.

Burp your baby often to expel the extra air he gulped while eating. This will keep the amount of tummy problems, spit-up, and hence laundry, to a minimum.

If your let down is painful, relax though the pain. The stiffer you are, the more painful it'll be. This is a good time to use your Lamaze breathing. It may not have done squat for your labor pains, but it might help now.

As the weeks pass, your body will adjust to your baby's needs, and it will slow down your production of milk. In the meantime, wear plenty of breast pads, push down on your nipples to stop the flow during embarrassing moments, and spread the wealth by donating your extra breast milk to a hospital NICU ward. (To find a needy hospital near you, see the appendix at the back of this book.) After all, a mind, and an overabundance of breast milk, is a terrible thing to waste.

Tongue Tied

Sometimes you look at your newborn and your heart fills with so much love that it actually hurts. Other times, your baby can cause pain in a different part of your anatomy: specifically, your nipples. If you find nursing to be hard on your nipples despite everything you try, there may be another reason for the pain. To find the source of the problem, you may not have to look any further than your baby's tongue.

Once in awhile, a baby is born with a short frenulum, that part of your body that you never quite knew the name of before. It's the plastic-tip-at-the-end-your-shoelace part of the body. A frenulum is the thin strip of membrane that's located underneath your tongue that attaches it to the floor of your mouth. When a baby has a short frenulum, it can cause incredible pain to your nipples when he latches on. Not only will you hurt, but your child may not get enough milk to drink since his tongue can't properly be placed behind your areola.

It's hard to tell just by looking if your newborn's tongue is frenulumly challenged. Instead, look for other signs. Does he make clucking sounds when he nurses? Is he unable to stick his tongue out past his lower gum? When he cries, do the sides of his tongue curl downward instead of forming a trough? Do his ears hang low and wobble to and fro? If he exhibits any of these traits, see a lactation specialist or your pediatrician (or a plastic surgeon, if he has the ear thing going on).

Once diagnosed, a short frenulum can be easily treated. It won't be pretty, but at least it'll be easy. That's because in order to rectify the situation, your pediatrician will need to actually clip the membrane. I know this sounds completely disgusting and gives new meaning to the term, "Man, that's nasty," but I swear, the pain is minimal—to your baby at least. You on the other hand will feel sick to your stomach watching it being cut. Fortunately, a newborn's frenulum is very frail. There should be little discomfort and only a couple of drops of blood, if any.

Oftentimes, however, a pediatrician will actually refuse to cut a baby's frenulum. He may feel that over time, the frenulum will soften up like a new pair of jeans. That of course is easy for *him* to say, since it's not his nipples that feel like they're put through a paper shredder every two hours. If your pediatrician refuses to do the old snip-snip, call a lactation specialist. These specialists can often recommend a pediatrician who is willing to do the procedure.

> "When my baby had a short frenulum, my pediatrician
> wouldn't cut it, so my lactation person wrote down the
> number of a pediatrician who would. When I saw him, I had
> to slip him $100 before he'd cut it. I felt like it was the
> forties and I was getting an illegal abortion."
>
> —Elizabeth

If your baby has a short frenulum, this snipping procedure will change your life. You'll find that once your baby's frenulum is snipped, the heavens will part and the pain will instantly disappear. If your baby had trouble gaining weight in the past, he'll start packing on the pounds like Renée Zellweger does before a *Bridget Jones* sequel. Not only will your baby be plumper, but he'll no doubt be happier, too, for a well-fed baby is a happy baby whether he's four weeks or forty years old.

Chapter 4

Feeding Frustrations

Okay. You've gotten past the pain of the early weeks of nursing. Your nipples are healing, your engorgement has settled down, and you finally got your husband to stop asking for a taste of your breast milk. But, as you can tell by the length of this book, there are still plenty of nursing hurdles to go.

For the past nine months, you've dealt with nothing but hurdles: morning sickness, sciatica, Braxton Hicks, and labor. Then came the bloody nipples, breast clogs, and figuring out how to work that damn breast pump. You pray that the challenges are behind you and that you can finally relax and enjoy this whole parenting thing. But *noooooo.* It seems that there are a boatload of challenges in store for you in the future. The good news is that most of these next nursing challenges aren't painful—not *physically* painful, that is.

I know you may be at the end of your rope and the bottom of your tube of nipple cream. You may even feel like throwing in the burp cloth and calling it a day on your nursing career. But if you know what problems to expect, and how to deal with them, you are far more likely to overcome them and stick with the program. Some of these awaiting nursing problems may be familiar to you. Others, like how nursing can make you feel like a virgin again during sex, may come as a complete surprise. So here's to education, some helpful ideas, and a few more vats of that nipple cream.

Growing, Growing, Groan!

You've been home for a few weeks and things are finally settling down. The visitors have stopped invading your home, and you can once again sit on a toilet seat without fear. Your kid has settled into a predicable eating routine of chowing down every two to three hours. Yes, besides the constant exhaustion and inability to remember things like your ATM number and your middle name, life is good.

But then your baby throws a curve ball that knocks you off your feet. For some inexplicable reason, your kid is eating more often than you did when you finally went off that no-carb diet! Now, instead of chowing down every two to three hours, he wants to eat every single hour around the clock! That's day and night, people! What the heck is going on here? Is your milk supply running low? Does your kid have a tapeworm? Why is he eating with the vim and vigor of a pie-eating contest winner?

The answer, my dear confused, frustrated friend, is that your baby is going through a growth spurt, a short period of time marked by incredible hunger. It usually occurs when your child is going through a stage of fast growth or increased physical activity, like learning how to turn over, crawl, or walk. Most growth periods last only about two or three days, but they seem to last much longer since you're up feeding your kid around the clock like a waitress at an all-night café.

Most growth spurts occur at more or less regular intervals. That's why it's a good idea to mark the dates on your calendar—just like your hubby did with your PMS so he knew when to wear his protective cup. The dates to circle are when your baby turns eight days, two weeks, four weeks, three months, four months, and six months old. Obviously, this is only an estimate since your baby isn't equipped with Swiss timing accuracy. These growth spurts continue from infancy through adolescence, but they go pretty much unnoticed after the first six months. That's because he'll most likely be eating solid food by then, and it's not very physically taxing to give him a few more spoonfuls of mashed peas.

During a growth spurt, you may think of supplementing your ravenous eater with formula (hell, you may think of supplementing him with a Hungry Man dinner), but try not to cave. Your breasts work on supply and demand, not unlike the incredible real estate boom of late, and should have plenty of milk available.

Yes, these growth spurts can be a great frustration to new moms and old moms alike, but you will get through them. Just think of the positives. Your baby is thriving. He's doing just what Mother Nature intended him to do. And, best of all, you get to eat even more calories just to keep up with the demand! Hello, cookie dough ice cream!

Baby Fat

There are several myths in life. There's the one that says you can't get pregnant the first time you have sex. There's the one that says you won't get a hangover if you drink only vodka. And the one that says if you breastfeed, you'll be back to your prepregnancy weight faster than you can say, "La Leche League." Well, I'm sorry to inform you that, just like the first two, this last myth is as fake as Pamela Anderson's chest.

Sure, there are some women whose bodies snap back after delivery. They credit this miracle to the fact that they exclusively breastfed their babies. But who's to say that their bodies wouldn't have snapped back if they didn't? Some women are born with incredible genes, which explains why they look so incredible *in* their jeans not long after giving birth.

True, there is some logic behind their reasoning. For one thing, it is proven that breastfeeding helps one certain part of your body return back to its normal: your uterus. When your baby sucks at your breast, your body releases the hormone oxytocin, which in turn makes your uterus cramp up and shrink down. So yes, if you want your uterus to be so tight you can bounce a quarter off of it, then by all means, nurse away.

In addition, if you breastfeed, you're body burns an additional 500 to 750 calories per day. In theory, that sounds like a weight watcher's dream. But the flaw behind this theory is that when your body burns more calories, your body screams for it to be fed. And we all know how persuasive our bodies can be when it comes to getting their way. Just see who wins out when it's just you and an open bag of Cool Ranch Doritos.

When it comes right down to it, your body's main goal is to keep itself alive, and over millions of years of evolution, it's become an expert at this task. It's learned to run from harm, get a fever when it's sick to battle infection, and not argue back when some whack job steals its parking spot. So it's no mystery why our bodies want to hold onto fat when we nurse. It knows that we need more calories in order to produce milk, so it clings to fat like a desperate woman clings to a bad boy.

I know that you're getting frustrated carrying around some of the extra weight you gained during your pregnancy. I know how it feels when strangers continue to ask when your baby is due. And I know how frustrating it is to have to buy yet another wardrobe of transitional clothing when you haven't even finished paying off your maternity wear.

But fret not. I can assure you that if you're one of the many women who is having trouble losing your "baby fat" while you nurse, there is still plenty of hope. For it may not be until you *stop* nursing that the weight will begin to fall off. Many, many women are finally able to be successful losing weight when they remove their babies from their boobs. Within weeks of weaning, they notice that their bodies start shriveling up like a contestant on *The Biggest Loser.*

Don't get me wrong. I'm not saying that your body will ever go back to exactly what it looked like before you conceived. Most women will always have a thicker waistline, as well as back fat that lingers like a visit from their in-laws. And let's not even talk about your vagina, which may look a bit like it suffered from a stroke. But if you diet and exercise, you stand a good chance of losing the weight. Keeping it off, I haven't been able to figure out yet, given that with kids comes a kitchen full of creamy mac and cheese and adorable animal crackers. But I'll cross my fingers that you can find a way.

So, if you keep seeing your closet full of preconception clothes just waiting to be worn again, don't get discouraged. Realize that this block of time in your life, when you're nursing, isn't about getting you back into shape. It's about keeping your baby healthy. And that's far more important than being able to wear your clingy knit dress! Besides, with a baby at home, why would you need to wear such a fancy dress anyway?

Sexual Healing

After your baby is born, your vagina is tired. It's been stretched and cut and stitched and bruised beyond recognition. It looks like genital road kill. Fortunately, your good doctor has given it a six-week sabbatical when it can relax, unwind, and be pampered with ice packs and sitz baths.

But after those six glorious weeks are over, it's time for it to get down to business. That's because after your forty-two-day respite, your long-denied husband is going to be all over you like white on rice (or "brown on rice," for those of you who are into the whole-grain kick). Even if your vagina has had time to heal its aching wounds, sex may still not be a pleasant experience since breastfeeding will add a level of pain to it that rivals any cherry-popping incident of years past.

The reason is that when you're breastfeeding, your body is still high on hormones, and these hormones tend to dry out your vagina and make the walls thin out. Because of this, penetration may be painful and feel like an internal rug burn. Even if you use a lot of lubrication and drink a lot of chardonnay, it can still be uncomfortable. Be sure to talk with your partner so that he can make the proper adjustments. Although he's as raring to go as a rodeo pony, he may have to pull in his reins and take things slowly at first. In time, as your hormones level off, things will ease up. But even though the pain of sex will be gone, there are other variables at work that can get in the way and take the love out of love making:

Exhaustion. When it comes to having sex, it takes a lot to get us women in the mood. We need a proper balance of foreplay, flattering words, and good lighting. But when we're suffering from total exhaustion, no amount of heavy petting, "I love you's," or candlelight is enough. After a full day of baby duty, combined with a only few hours of sleep, the last thing we want to do is to get our hearts racing. We get enough of that during the day, when we see the baby stop breathing for an instant.

You gave at the office . . . and at home. Having a baby is like giving birth to an eight-pound to-do list. Every moment of the day is filled with something to feed, wipe, bathe, or put down. If you work, this is on top of the endless things that need your attention at the office. At the end of the day, the last thing you want to deal with is yet another need to fill, even if that need is one of your husband's.

You've already been felt up enough for the day, thank you very much. We women are tactile creatures. We love holding hands and getting massages. But too much of a good thing can feel downright irritating. That's why after a full day of having your body be groped by your baby, you have no desire to have it be groped by your spouse.

Leaky breasts. Boobs leak. Especially during the first few months of breastfeeding. And being sexually aroused makes them leak even more. Once you see your breasts spurt milk all over your husband, the only desire you have is to laugh, or maybe cry, or in some cases, both. My advice, don't be on top unless you want to douse your husband like a small brush fire. Although if it gets him out of the mood, it may not be such a bad idea!

I Want My MTV (Medicine, Tobacco, & Vodka)!

I have a confession to make. I'm an addict. It's not an addiction to anything illegal or one that will lead to an unflattering mug shot, but it is an addiction nonetheless. What am I addicted to, you may ask? It's that wonderful "fixes everything so I can rest", medicine. Sure it's green and it tastes like crap, but when I have a cold, it's a liquid slice of heaven. If you have an addiction to any substance that's forbidden while you nurse, it can make your nursing experience quite a struggle to deal with.

"I had a jalapeño pizza for lunch the other day,

and my baby and I were belching at the same time."

—Susan

As all you good lactating mamas know, ingesting medications or toxins when you're nursing is a big fat no-no. When milk is flowing through your bosom, you have to live a life as clean and proper as Mary Ellen Walton's (or Donna Martin's, for you younger kids). To some degree, you must deny yourself some of the best things that life has to offer, like caffeine, alcohol, tobacco, certain foods, and yes drugs, which includes my beloved green liquid-gold medicine. You've just spent nine long months avoiding these things when you were pregnant. How long are you expected to live like a one-dimensional television character?

For the most part, dietary restrictions during nursing are far less severe than those you had during pregnancy. In fact, your doctor may tell you that you don't really have to change your diet at all when you're breastfeeding. You can actually have limited amounts of caffeine and alcohol. And the ban that was in place during pregnancy on foods like soft imported cheeses and raw foods like fish, seafood, and meat have all been lifted. But if you're like some moms, you don't want to take any chances. Even if there's not enough bacteria to harm your baby, you don't want to risk getting yourself sick. Life is hard enough right now without contracting *E. coli*, thank you very much.

On the other hand, if your baby has colic, you have not only my sincere condolences but a lengthy list of foods to abstain from as well. That's because certain foods may irritate colic and make your baby cry more than Tiger Woods does when he wins the Masters. Some of the top culinary culprits are wheat, eggs, nuts, shellfish, citrus, dairy, and gassy veggies.

While you breastfeed, many prescription medications will be banned as well. And that includes your birth control pills. Sure, you may not be having your period now, but that doesn't mean that there isn't a nubile egg right now ready and waiting for a broad-shouldered sperm to come her way. But birth control pills are made up of hormones, and those hormones can lower your milk production. A diaphragm is a good alternative, but if you used one before you conceived, be sure to have it resized. It seems that pregnancy may increase not only your belt size but your diaphragm size as well.

Between your pregnancy and your nursing, you're tired of living a clean and wholesome life. You've spent the first decades on the planet just growing old enough to enjoy these pleasures. But take a breath and relax. Realize that you won't be nursing forever. And in the meantime, this wholesome life is keeping your body at its best so that it can deal with the demands of parenthood. So, until its time to wean, put that drink down, that cigarette out, that medicine cap on, and your legs closed (until you get yourself a proper form of birth control).

Nip/Stuck

There's a drama in the breastfeeding world that's more intense than any *Law & Order* episode ever was. It's a drama about nipple confusion, and it happens when your little one confuses your soft, warm nipple for the rubbery hard nipple of a bottle. He'll become frustrated by the various options, not unlike how we feel choosing between PCs and Macs. Once confused, he may go with the easiest option of the bottle and give up nursing entirely. (Cue dramatic music: da da da dum!)

The reason for this is simple. Not only do the nipples on the bottle and breast differ, but the way that milk is expressed from them does as well. Throw in the nipple of a pacifier, where your baby sucks and gets no liquid reward, and you've got yourself one confused camper.

Not all newborns experience nipple confusion. Some have no trouble dealing with any nipple that's thrown in their mouths. But others do. That's because breastfeeding is a far more complex feat to master than bottlefeeding. With breastfeeding, the baby has to learn how to open his mouth wide, put your nipple deep inside his mouth, and then use his gums to literally milk you like a cow, drawing the milk out from back to front.

Bottlefeeding, on the other hand, is the lazy way to eat because gravity does most of the work for your baby. He doesn't have to close his tongue and mouth around your nipple to form a seal that rivals a zip-lock container. Nor does he have to worry about his tongue and gums forming the proper sucking action. In fact, he can just kick back and suck with only his lips.

If you'd rather be safe than stressed, consider nursing exclusively for the first three to four weeks (that means no bottles *or* pacifiers). By doing this, you will give your baby time to master the most challenging way to suck first, after which he can be introduced to the easier ways. It's like learning to drive a stick shift before learning an automatic or learning how to have sex before you can just lie there and go over your to-do list in your head.

If you introduce bottles before this time frame, you run the risk of having your baby nurse you in the same way he would suck from a bottle. When that happens, your nipples become shredded like an incriminating White House document. On the other hand, if you wait too long to introduce a bottle or pacifier, you run the risk of having your baby refuse to take it all together. This of course makes going back to work, or leaving your kid with a sitter to regain your sanity, quite impossible.

Personally, I've never seen a case of nipple confusion, and I think it may be one of those old wives' tales. Besides, if your baby ever starts refusing to take your breasts after you've introduced a bottle, you can always retrain him. At this young age, kids are as malleable as pizza dough. If your baby is refusing to take your breast after taking a bottle, follow these simple rules, and life as you knew it will slowly return:

- **Put a temporary ban on artificial nipples.** If for some reason you need your child to ingest something other than breast milk, use an eyedropper, a small cup, or a spoon.
- **Pump or express until your milk is flowing before you start nursing.** That way your baby will experience the joy of instant gratification that he gets from using a bottle.
- **At first, retrain when your baby when he's calm (but not hungry), usually at night or first thing in the morning.** You don't want to stress out an already stressed-out kid.
- **Before your baby latches on, remind him to open his mouth wide by opening your mouth wide as well.** Babies are like annoying little siblings and copy everything you do.

Pumping Problems

I was never a good pumper. You'd think that having breasts large enough to reach from one zip code to another would mean I could pump enough to feed a third-world country. But instead I would pump for days and barely get enough milk to feed a baby squirrel. In addition, I never quite understood how the whole pumping process worked. If I pumped, wouldn't I be taking milk away from my baby? And when was the best time to pump? Before feedings? During? After? Plus, if I pumped, wouldn't I just be telling my body to produce more milk, which would cause my bloated boobs to burst like an overfilled water balloon? Between my low output and my confusion, I resigned to the fact that my breasts could never be away from my baby for more than a two-hour stretch.

That's why, when doing research for this section, I turned to an expert in the field: Corkey Harvey, RN, MS, certified lactation counselor, and co-owner of the Pump Station in Los Angeles. Her first rule of thumb when it comes to pumping is that there are no absolutes. Yes, there are guidelines to follow, but in the end, do what works best for you.

The first guideline is to get yourself a good pump. I made the mistake of buying a cheap manual pump in order to save money. With it I barely got any milk at all, although I did get rock-hard biceps from the workout. Check your insurance policy. Some smart companies cover breast pumps since they know it'll save them money down the line due to fewer baby illnesses. If your insurance doesn't cover the expense, get the best pump you can afford, ideally a double pump so you can pump in half the time.

Guideline number two is that you should pump in the morning because that's when your breasts are the most full. Wait a half hour after you've finished nursing and then give pumping a try. Adjust the pump so it's on the strongest level you can tolerate without feeling pain. Don't expect the milk to come squirting out of you like Old Faithful. The pump isn't nearly as effective at bringing down and expressing milk as your baby's mouth. Resist the temptation to stare at your nipple every second awaiting the milk to come down. As they say, a watched nipple never spurts.

If you're not producing much milk or you're having trouble with let down, pump one breast while your baby nurses with the other. That way your baby will bring down the milk. You can also try nursing your baby on one side, then, when he switches over to the other, pump the side he just finished to get any good stuff that was left inside.

If pumping only in the morning doesn't give you your quota of milk, pump a half hour after another feeding as well. Just remember to pump at the same time every day so your body will learn to produce more milk at that time. Keep in mind that as the day progresses, your body naturally produces less milk to correspond with your kid's late afternoon/early evening fussy time, when he wants to be stuck on you like a tattoo.

When you pump, be safe. Wash and dry your hands thoroughly. Clean the various pumping parts well in hot, soapy water (or put them through the dishwasher, if the instructions recommend it) and be sure to dry them thoroughly. Also, check that the breast shield you're using is the right size for your nipple so that you're comfortable . . . well, as comfortable as you can be with a motorized contraption juicing you like an orange.

Once you finish pumping, store the container in the fridge during the day. You can add milk to it later on from subsequent pumping sessions; just wait for the fresh milk to cool down before adding it to the original bottle. You don't want to add warm milk to cool milk. If you're going to freeze it, be sure not to overfill the bottles or storage bags. Liquid expands when it freezes, and few things are worse than going through all that hell to make a bottle only to have it explode in your freezer like a can of soda. It's enough to make you hate your husband. So what if he had nothing to do with it. You're going to hate your husband a lot during these early days of motherhood for no apparent reason.

Be familiar with storage rules and regulations so that your stored breast milk is safe to drink. You're basically turning your bottle of breast milk into a petri dish with a nipple if you don't follow these guidelines:

"I finally had a large enough stockpile of pumped bottles in the freezer to go back to work. Then we had a power outage and I had to put them in a cooler and race to get to a nearby relative's house before they were ruined. I felt like I was delivering an organ to a needy transplant patient."

—Kate

- **Breast milk can be kept at room temperature for four hours.** It can be refrigerated for five to seven hours and frozen for six to twelve months.
- **Once the milk is thawed, it must be used right away.** Never refreeze!
- **To thaw frozen milk,** place it in the refrigerator overnight, or hold the bottle or plastic bag under running water, or put it in a warm bowl of water for about twenty minutes.
- **Never microwave breast milk, because the process can change the makeup of the milk.** More importantly, it can create hot spots, which could burn your baby's mouth. Parenting is hard enough without dealing with your baby's mouth blisters. (You can also use a bottle warmer once it's thawed).

If you need further help or information about pumping, contact a lactation specialist. You can find them in hospitals or breastfeeding centers, or you can check your local phone book. (See the resources listed in the appendix at the back of this book for more ideas.) I know I've said it before, but these specialists are wonderful. They know everything there is about nursing, and that includes the proper practice of the pump.

Take Your Show on the Road

As time goes by, you've become adept at breast-feeding. Your pumping skills are sublime, your baby latches on with perfection, and your milk comes down with the ease of a debutante on a spiral staircase. With your new inner confidence, you finally feel the urge to venture back into the land of the living, and shoe sales, once again. But unless you want to rush home every couple of hours to feed your kid, you have to learn how to take your show, and your nipples, on the road.

Breastfeeding in public can be very intimidating. You've seen women do it with the grace of an Olympic skater. They hold their babies in one hand and their moccacinos in the other, somehow managing to get themselves undressed and the babies latched on without skipping a beat—or spilling their coffee.

But for you, the whole process seems so unnatural. Whipping your boob out in a crowded place goes against everything you've been told since

the day you could fill out a tube top. Besides,
how do you even go about doing it? Is there a
trick to disrobing? An art of a blind latch? And
won't your kid suffocate under your shirt without
any fresh air? The whole thing is more confusing
than remembering which way to set your clock
during daylight savings time.

The amount of difficulty you'll have nursing in public will be in direct proportion to your
personal modesty level. I find that many women
who survive pregnancy and childbirth are far less
modest than those who haven't gone through it.
There's nothing like nine months of embarrassing and uncontrollable bodily functions followed
by a day of lying spread eagle in front of an audience, all while pushing out what feels like the
largest bowel movement of your life, to rid you
of your modesty.

If performing a personal act like nursing in
public and stripping in front of a crowd provokes
panic, relax. Remember, practice makes perfect.
Before you take your show on the road, do what
you did when you learned how to dance: Practice
in front of the mirror. Sit down in front of a full-
length mirror with your baby in your arms, and
give it go while checking yourself out. See what
body parts play peek-a-boo as you slip your kid

under your shirt, unhook your bra, and get him latched on. Once you're confident that you can pull it off without committing a wardrobe malfunction, give it a go.

To help steady your nerves, here are some tips about how to nurse in public without committing indecent exposure:

- **The first time you try it, take a good friend along.** She can provide moral support (as well as additional screening to block out the crowd).
- **Bring something with you to drape over your body before you whip out your boob.** A lightweight receiving blanket is an excellent choice and makes a great protective shield.
- **Wear a nursing bra that's easy to snap and unsnap.** Look for one that you can operate with only one hand. I know this will take some practice, but people have learned to paint by holding the brush in their teeth, so we're all capable of many things.
- **Until you're more comfortable, wear nursing shirts that are designed with slits to get your breasts in and out of there in the most modest way possible.**

Later you can try a button-down shirt, but
remember to unbutton it from the bottom
to make a "shirt tent."

- **Nurse in a sling.** The sling has high walls,
  so it's difficult for anyone to enjoy the show.
  If you don't have a sling, you can try to
  nurse in your Baby Björn. It's surprisingly
  discreet, and you can nurse on the go. (Just
  make sure that your baby is heavy enough
  to meet the lower weight limit before putting him inside.)

- **Don't set yourself up for failure by
  wearing a dress.** There ain't no way to get
  a baby under there without showing more
  skin than a cage dancer.

Keep in mind that no matter how adept you
become at nursing in public, people will always
stare at you. But that doesn't mean they'll look
at you with disgust. Some women stare because
they're remembering what it was like when they
nursed. Some men stare because they're fanta-
sizing about sucking on a boob and having beer
come out. And yes, there will be others who stare
at you in disapproval, but just ignore those people
like you do the ones who try to douse you with
perfume when you enter a department store.

Stressed Out!

Having a new baby can be a very stressful time. You're up all night. You don't seem to have a minute to yourself. And you fight with your spouse all day (no, it's not just you). If you choose to breastfeed, you're adding yet another layer of stress to the seventeen-layer cake of stress that's already your life.

One layer of stress stems from that fact that, unless you have a stockpile of frozen bottles at your disposal, you can't be away from your baby for more than a few hours. Because of this, you're forced to take your baby with you to run errands, which, as you quickly learn, is a pain in the ass. When you have a baby by your side, there's no such thing as popping into a store. Not only do you have to deal with your kid, but you also have to haul around the various accoutrements that come along with him, like the stroller, carrier, and fully stocked diaper bag that's equipped to deal with any bodily function emergency. If you don't bring your kid along, however, you're stressed that you'll get into an accident while you're out, and if your boobs aren't home in time to feed him, your baby will die of dehydration. (No, that's not just you, either.)

Another layer of stress is that you can't feel good in anything you wear. The buttons of your shirts pull and everything you own is inevitably stained with baby puke. You also worry about leaking in public. Between your breasts dripping with milk and your crotch dripping with lochia, you're a walking Tivoli fountain!

You're also stressed because your house is falling apart. You haven't cleaned it in weeks, there's no food in the fridge, the houseplants are on their last leaves, and the only thing stacked higher than your unpaid bills is your pile of dirty laundry. I bet if you applied, your house could qualify for a FEMA loan.

Your baby is stressing you out as well. After almost nonstop nursing sessions, you're sick of your kid grabbing at your chest and staring at it like a prepubescent boy. You're not sure if he loves you for you or for the fact that your boobs are like a twenty-four-hour soft-serve dispenser.

If you have older children, you're stressed because you never have time to sit down and nurse when you have an active toddler to care for—a toddler who can't do anything without you, like tie his shoe, blow his nose, or read *The Big Green Monster* for the zillionth time that day. And a toddler can out-scream your infant by 100 decibels if you refuse his requests. Sure, one day he'll be able to comprehend that you're busy and will be with him shortly, but for now, you have a better chance of teaching him how to share . . . and that's saying something!

I know nursing is hard. And I know that life with a baby can be so hard on its own. But before you turn in your worn-out boobs for a fresh-off-the-showroom-floor bottle of formula, here are some ideas to make your nursing life easier. Granted, you shouldn't expect miracles. Until your kid drives off to college, your life is going to be as mad and hectic as the floor of the New York Stock Exchange. But at least these ideas may take some of the edge off:

- **Make a nursing kit.** Get a basket or a bucket and fill it with everything you need by your side while you nurse. These items include such things as your nursing log, a pen, the remote control, a cordless phone, address book, gift catalogs, a bottle of water, and snacks.
- **Get some cute nursing shirts.** This may be a challenge because nursing women are a fairly ignored bunch by clothing designers. When you're pregnant, there are plenty

of stylish clothes to choose from, but now that you're a mom, it's hard not to look, and feel, frumpy. Until Old Navy and Banana Republic come out with nursing lines, you'll just have to go on the Internet and let your fingers do the walking. (Check out the resources listed in the appendix at the back of this book for some Web sites that cater to nursing moms.)

- **Supplement.** If you're a good pumper, supplement with a bottle so that your husband can help out with at least one feeding while you rest. A few extra hours of continuous sleep can make a world of difference to your mental well-being. If you're not a good pumper, dare I say, use formula at night. (I know I'll get a protest call from the La Leche League, but I'm sticking with my call. In my opinion, losing your sanity is far worse than giving your kid a bottle of formula.)

- **Get support!** Seek out parenting groups, mommy and me groups, or nursing groups—or else you'll soon be seeking support from an AA group.

Chapter 5

"Express" Yourself

If you're going back to work and want to continue feeding your baby breast milk, I applaud you. In the world of nursing, there's nothing more challenging than having to deal with pumping at the office. It's the triple gainer with a twist of breastfeeding. Your blissful life of holding your warm cuddly muffin and sharing some one-on-one time will be traded in for having to lock yourself in a cold, sterile bathroom and bonding with an electrical appliance.

Despite the challenge, millions of courageous women tackle this feat five days a week, month after month, and they come out gold medal winners. They face the obstacles and are awarded the prize of bottles of liquid gold so they can continue to feed their babies the healthiest food on Earth. Isn't mother's love the best?

But what are some of the obstacles that women face when they pump at work? And how does one begin to deal with them? That, my soon-to-be-lactating-at-the-office friend, is the topic of this chapter. It is chock full of "how to's" and "what shoulds" and "Who can I kill for making it so difficult to earn a living while feeding my baby?" In sum, it's the perfect chapter to read before punching that time clock once again.

Fortunately, you can do plenty of things to make returning to work easier, and many of them can be done before you even return. Like anything else in life, it's good to be prepared. You should carry a cell phone in case of emergencies. Wear clean underwear in case you're in an accident. Keep the number of a Domino's Pizza place handy when you attempt to cook that meal that looked so easy when Emeril did it. And finally, when it comes to pumping at the office, you should know what problems to expect so you can deal with them when they rear their ugly heads.

As you know, if you don't pump often at work, your milk supply will dwindle. Then you won't be able to pump enough milk, and you'll have to supplement with formula. This in turn means that your baby won't need to eat as often, since formula is more filling, so you'll produce even less milk. Before you know it, your breasts will be empty, and your cabinets will be full . . . of formula, that is.

Bear in mind that although it's difficult, the majority of problems that come with pumping at work occur only for a short time. In the beginning, you'll have to pump the most. Then, when your baby starts eating solid food, your time at the pump will be far less. Until then, expect frustrations, stick with the plan, and learn how to deal with the problems that occur while keeping your baby, and your 401(k), growing strong.

To Work, or Not to Work?
That Is the Financial Question

Some women are totally confident about their decision to return to work after they have their babies. Either they have fulfilling careers that bring them much joy, or they just need the dough. But then, as their maternity leaves come to an end, they question their decision. They gaze at their beautiful babies and can't imagine saying goodbye to their li'l snookums five days a week to rejoin the rat race.

If you're finding it impossible to return to work, you may want to go back to the drawing board. Maybe the joys of motherhood far exceed the joys of corporate-hood. If you're lucky enough to be able to live on only your husband's income, the decision to stay at home is easy. But if you can't, and you're planning to return to work to help pay the bills, take a moment to factor in all the variables and expenses. On the surface, having a weekly paycheck seems to keep your bank account in the black, but there are hidden expenses of returning to work that you may not have considered.

For instance, did you take into account the skyrocketing cost of child care? How about the expense of daily lunches at restaurants rather than eating sandwiches at home? Did you factor in the cost of buying a new wardrobe of transitional work clothes and the price of having them dry cleaned? What about the expense of makeup and having your hair done in that "climbing the corporate ladder" look? Did you add in the cost of gas and wear and tear on your car for your daily commute? On that note, did you call your auto insurance carrier to see what kind of savings you're entitled to if you're a stay-at-home mom?

What about the price of the breast pump itself, along with the necessary storage bags, sterilizers, bottles, and warmers? Will you need a house-keeper to take over the chores that you won't be able to manage during the day? By the time you've paid for these hidden expenses, your big paycheck may not be so big after all.

Also, did you go through your bills and see where you could cut costs? Do you really need all those cable channels? Or Internet access on your cell phone? Can you cancel the daily paper and give up your Starbucks latte? What about color-ing your hair every other time yourself and only going out to eat once a month instead of once a week? Individually, these expenses may not be much, but when you add them all together, these, plus the many more you can either cut or trim, may be the difference between staying home and going to the office.

Going back to work may not be an all-or-nothing situation. Many companies provide job sharing so you and a coworker who also has time restraints can split one job. Or, with the help of modern-day technology and a lot of unsightly electric cords, you can bring your projects home and work on them when your baby naps. Or you can go into the office for important things like department-head meetings and free bagels in the lunch room.

So if you're second-guessing your decision to return to work full time, do the math. Then talk to your boss and see if there's any flexibility in your position. Remember, the squeaky wheel gets the grease, and in this case, it may also get you more time with your baby. And that may be the best situation for both your bank account and your mental well-being.

The Truth about Maternity Leave

While you're still at home pondering your decision to return to work, let's talk a moment about the confusion that surrounds maternity leave. Sure, the United States is a wonderful place to live if you're into things like free speech and Thanksgiving, but it sucks when it comes to taking time off from work to spend with your baby. Unlike many other developed countries, there is no such thing as guaranteed paid maternity leave. Some companies offer six weeks of paid leave. Some guarantee that your job will be protected for twelve weeks, and some even allow your spouse to take leave as well. But others, especially smaller companies or those where you haven't worked for very long or only work part time, guarantee absolutely nothing. That's why it's important to talk to your employer (or human resources department) about the regulations at your specific company before you venture into that labor room so you know what to expect when you come out.

Even though the laws aren't great when it comes to maternity leave, things are getting better. The Family and Medical Leave Act (knows as the FMLA for those in the legal biz) was passed in 1993. It guarantees that *most* workers can take up to twelve weeks of leave after a birth or an adoption and still have a job waiting for them at the other end. I say "most" because the law isn't universal and doesn't cover many smaller companies. Also, just to be clear, the law doesn't entitle employers to *pay* you for those twelve weeks. The FMLA provides only that you're guaranteed to have your job back when you return (or a similar job with the same pay and seniority).

The laws can be confusing, and they vary from state to state and company to company. That's why the length and security of your maternity leave will vary if you've worked for years as a federal employee in Sacramento or as a weekend bartender in St. Louis. But no matter where you live or what type of company you work for, there are ways to increase the amount of time you can take off from work. One is to consider getting short-term disability insurance (which covers maternity leave) through your company or private insurance. You can also take vacation days, personal time, and sick days, which you've hopefully stockpiled like Cipro during the anthrax scare of years past.

So speak up, know your rights, and plan ahead (ideally when you're still pregnant so you can accrue those sick days and vacation time). Who knows? Maybe because you're being more assertive, and if you're pregnant, because you outweigh your boss by fifty pounds, you'll be able to get whatever you want.

Home Work

No matter how much maternity leave you'll be able to take, there are plenty of things you can do at home to make your transition back to work a smoother one. Yes, I know that right now you're busy enough filling out baby logs, assembling baby products, and feeding more hungry visitors than the Hard Rock Cafe, but try to fit them in. True, one of the most important things you can do at home is to master breastfeeding so you can build up a good milk supply. Not only will this give you plenty of milk to feed your baby, you'll also have plenty of milk to pump later on. But once you get that established, try to get as many of the following things done as possible, too:

1. **After three weeks of strict breastfeeding, introduce a bottle to your baby.** Avoid doing this any sooner since it could lead to "nipple confusion." Much later, and it could lead to your baby refusing to take the bottle altogether. When it's time to introduce a bottle, have someone else do it. Your baby wasn't born yesterday (okay, a few days shy of that), and he knows full well that you're the one with the goods. He may want the drink directly from the well instead of some plastic replica thereof. (For tips, see "Nip/Stuck" on page 112.)

2. **Become BFFs with your breast pump.** Going back to work will be stressful enough without having to figure out how to operate your pump. Besides, becoming a proficient pumper will take some time, and some frustrations, and it's best not to have to deal with them with coworkers looking

over your shoulder . . . or down your dress. Besides, pumping at home for a couple of weeks will give you a good supply of frozen bottles!

3. **Get your office clothes in order.** If you're not back in your prepregnancy wardrobe by the time you go back to work (and who is, except celebrities who have trainers, personal chefs, and upcoming red-carpet moments), you'll need to buy, or borrow, some appropriate pumping clothes. (See "Dress to Express" on page 152 for more specifics.)

4. **Find out exactly where you'll be pumping at the office.** This way, you can get the necessary accoutrements. You may need a cooler, an extension cord, a privacy sign, a folding table, or some other special equipment to be comfortable. Also, know in advance where you can store these things, as well as your pump, breast pads, a few extra shirts in case of leaking, storage bags, and cleaning supplies for your pump. Who knows, with all that crap, you may even get a bigger office out of the deal!

5. **Find good child care.** Ideally, this should be done when you're pregnant since finding

a quality person to care for your baby is more difficult than finding a bathing suit that makes you feel good. Do lots of research, and get plenty of references. If you're looking for a day-care facility, consider one that's close to your office so you can drop by to nurse on your lunch hour (and make surprise visits to check out how good they are when no one is looking). If you want someone to come to your home, consider hiring a person who drives so she can bring your baby to you for a daytime feeding. Or, in an ideal world, see if you can get enough people with young kids together at work so you can push for a day-care situation at the office.

6. **Practice giving the evil eye.** You'll need it for disapproving coworkers who may not agree with your decision to continue breastfeeding in a dignified, professional place like the office.

It's Just Emotions That're Making Me Crazy

My God, when will the roller-coaster ride of emotions ever end? Last year, it was the emotional turmoil of trying to conceive, when every month's unfertilized egg that passed through your loins brought on a river of tears. Then came the topsy-turvy ride of pregnancy, with its unending mood swings. Then came birth, when you experienced overwhelming hatred toward your spouse, then overpowering love for your beautiful baby. And now, every day since your baby has popped out of your oven, you've felt a mixture of joy, baby blues, and constant exhaustion. When will the madness end?

Unfortunately, it won't end any time soon, I'm afraid, especially if you're headed back to the office. Leaving your helpless baby at home goes against every maternal instinct you have. No matter how much your little one has fussed or cried or puked these past weeks, you will find leaving him unbearable. And no matter how much you trust your caregiver, how many great references or medical degrees she has, you'll worry that she'll be watching daytime television while your cat is taking its afternoon nap on your baby's head.

As your maternity leave comes to an end, it will get harder and harder to push the thought out of your mind that you'll be returning to work. You can't imagine leaving your ever-growing bundle of joy to face an ever-growing inbox. You can't fathom building your firm's client list while someone else is building a block tower with your baby. That's why, when the big day finally arrives, and you kiss your baby good-bye, you'll drive away feeling overwhelming guilt, sorrow, and (surprisingly) hunger, since the morning was so chaotic you forgot to eat any breakfast.

Just know that all of these emotions are perfectly normal. Going back to work after having a baby can be difficult. And as hard as you thought it would be, you end up wishing it were just that easy. At work, you'll miss the physical closeness you had with your baby and fear that you'll miss out on all the precious firsts. You'll have a hole in your heart that only your baby can fill, although you'll try to your dangedest to fill it with dough-nuts from the break room.

As hard as it may be, you must focus on the positives. You're not deserting your child so that you can spend the day at the spa. You're work-ing to keep a roof over your head and food in the fridge. You are a wonderful mom, which is why you feel so bad in the first place. If you *didn't* feel bad, then I'd worry. Besides, it's not as if you're leaving your baby with Britney Spears. Your baby is safe and secure with a family member, a qualified caretaker, or a facility that you've checked out thoroughly. By being with other people besides just you, your baby will get plenty of attention, socialization skills, and love.

No matter whether you leave your baby at home or in a day-care facility, see if you can hook up a Web cam so you can check on your baby throughout the day. Seeing firsthand that your baby is safe, snug, warm, and not being smothered by the cat can go a long way to relieving your worries. It will also make you more productive at work, since 40 percent of your brain won't be stressing about the welfare of your kid while the other 50 percent is trying to focus on work. (There's always about 10 percent of your brain that's thinking about the doughnuts in the break room.)

As the days and weeks pass, leaving your baby at home while you go to work will get easier. Sure, it may always tug on your heartstrings a little when you kiss your baby goodbye. But then, at the end of your day, when you're greeted by your baby's big smile and his bigger hug, you'll know that he's going to be okay. And when you're greeted by that big paycheck at that end of the week, you'll know that your bank account's going to be okay as well.

Can't It at Least Buy Me Dinner First?

In the beginning, pumping is a new and challenging experience. But then, like anything else you do over and over again, like cooking dinner or having sex with your husband, the novelty wears off. After a few weeks of pumping at the office, you'll develop a love/hate relationship with your breast pump that rivals the one you have with any sibling. You'll hate plugging it in and strapping it on and having it knead your breasts like an inexperienced lover.

These feelings will confuse you. How can you hate the contraption that's responsible for keeping your baby so healthy? Yet how can you not resent hooking yourself up to a wall jack every few hours? You feel like a prisoner. A leaky, engorged, constantly thirsty prisoner. No matter how busy your day is, or how many important phone calls you have to return, you still have to take time out every few hours to pump. If you don't pump as often as you nurse, you'll threaten your milk supply and risk getting clogs, mastitis, or worse. But if you do, you risk getting stared at by your coworkers, getting behind at work, and having your job threatened. Why is raising a kid so much harder on us moms? If men had to pump at the office, there'd be designated rooms with fifty-inch plasma screens and leather La-Z-Boys with heated seats.

If this is your current and resentful state of mind, chances are that pumping is taking you longer than it should. There are tricks to the breastfeeding trade that can speed up your pumping so you can get back to work. Trick number one is to get yourself a good pump. When it comes to pumps, you really do get what you pay for.

"When I looked for a pump, I didn't want to spend $300, so I bought a cheaper one for $150. After a few weeks, the pump broke and when I called the 800 number, I was told that this pump was only meant for occasional pumping. Then had to run to the store during my lunch break and buy that $300 pump after all. It's expensive to buy cheap."

—Sarah

Trick number two is to get your milk down fast. When dealing with a metal contraption instead of a warm, delicious-smelling baby, it may take longer for your milk to come down. This is especially true when you're pumping at the office. The business world is not the most conducive place to perform a private act (although millions have tried to sneak in quickies behind closed doors). Offices are filled with the stress of schedules and deadlines, so let down can be a struggle. If this happens, try to relax. Take a deep breath, look at a photo of your baby, and bring in a pair of his jammies to smell. If you have a portable music system like a Walkman or an iPod, load it up with relaxing tunes or even the lullaby that you play to your baby at bedtime. To take your mind off work, skim through parenting magazines instead of budget reports. This is your time to be a mother, not a member of the workforce.

After some time and practice, things will improve. Soon, your milk will go down as easy as a cold beer on a hot summer's day. And a good breast pump will get it out fast. In no time you'll be back at your desk dealing with the phone messages and the urgent e-mails you got while you were pumping, and then the only thing you'll resent is your job.

Working Conditions

Not only are some jobs better at providing health benefits and cake on employees' birthdays, they're also better at providing good pumping conditions. In the perfect scenario, you'd be allowed to take a break whenever you needed. You'd have a private office where you could pump without onlookers or embarrassment, a personal dishwasher for sterilization, and a small refrigerator by your side to store your milk. But unless your last name is Trump, Gates, or the same as the owner of your company, finding a job like that is nearly impossible.

As you know from personal experience, most working conditions are not as ideal. Many employees don't have their own offices, so they're forced to pump in the communal break room, bathroom, or supply closet. There are others who pump in their cubicles and struggle to drown out the sound of the distracting whir of the pump. Not every office is equipped with a refrigerator to store your milk, so you might have to beg the restaurant next door to use theirs and pray that an employee doesn't mistake it for coffee creamer. Even if you do have a fridge, it may be so far from where you pump that you have to scurry down the hall with your full bag and hope you don't bump into a coworker and burst it all over his Hugo Boss three piece.

"It was a long way from the private room where I pumped to the group freezer. Three times a day I'd have to carry my see-through bag down the hall and hope no one would stop me to chat because once they saw 'the bag,' they'd be totally grossed out. It was like I was carrying a bag full of boogers."

—Marjorie

There might not be a convenient outlet where you can plug your pump, so you may have to use an extension cord and hear coworkers curse as they trip over it. If you pump in the bathroom, you may not have anywhere to rest your pump, meaning you have to sit on the cold floor and stare at the tile. If your office doesn't have a dishwasher, steril-izing your breast pump and bottles will be quite a challenge. As you know, it's important to sterilize everything that goes into your infant's mouth since babies don't have strong immune systems. If there isn't a dishwasher available, you're forced to simply rinse and hope for the best.

These are but a fraction of the challenges you may be faced with when trying to pump at the office. And these are but a few of the solutions to those challenges:

- If your office doesn't come equipped with a dishwasher, get a microwave steriliz- ing kit. Most offices have a microwave, and if they don't, they're cheap to buy and can be kept near your desk. These microwave kits can sterilize breast pump parts, bottles, nipples, and caps in only a few minutes.

- If you work in a profession where you're on the road for a part of your day and away from a power source, get a battery operated pump. They're not as strong as electric models, and most can only pump one breast at a time, but in a pinch, it's certainly better than expressing your milk by hand!

- Make a privacy sign. If you're worried that someone will come in your office, cubicle, break room, or bathroom while you pump, and you want privacy, buy or make a sign. Something that has a drawing of a milking cow is always a favorite.

- If you don't have a refrigerator at work, store your bags of expressed milk in a cooler equipped with ice packs. And don't confuse coolers with those insulated bags that store both hot and cold foods. They're not nearly as effective.

- If you have a demanding job, a private office, and not a lot of time to pump, get a nursing halter. It's a contraption that keeps your hands free so you can pump and send an important e-mail at the same time. Or you can make your own nursing halter by taking a sports bra and cutting out holes for your areolas. When you stick your pump through the holes, your sports bra should keep the pump in place.

If you don't see a remedy for a specific problem you're having, be creative and think one up. Then you can package it, sell it, and become the newest mommy millionaire and say to hell with pumping at the office!

Dealing with Coworkers

Every job comes complete with coworkers who can make your life miserable. They spread office gossip, sabotage your work so they can get ahead, and eat your container of yogurt, even though it clearly has your name written on it. When you have to pump at the office, it gives your coworkers yet another reason to be in your face. That's because they see your mammary glands as two big "Get out of Work" signs, and they resent you for it.

Oftentimes these coworkers are jealous that you can take long sanctioned breaks in order to pump. You can step away from your desk any time you want, while they get sneers and dirty e-mails if they get back from their lunch hours five minutes late. And to make matters worse, they're the ones who are asked to cover your desk while you're away.

Coworkers also resent it if it's time for a meeting and they have to wait for you to finish pumping. They envision you behind closed doors attached to a pump while giving yourself a mani-pedi and listening to Sarah McLaughlin's latest album on your iPod. Little do they know that you're on the cold floor crying your eyes out because you can't get your milk to let down.

They may resent that the only place you have to pump is the common break room or bathroom, so they have to wait for you to finish before they can go in. No matter how cute your privacy sign may be, all your coworkers see is that they can't refill their morning cup of Joe or pee when they want. They may also lose their appetite when they open the door to the fridge and come face to face with your bags of steaming breast milk. To you it's no biggie, but to others, it's like staring at a baggie of poo.

If you notice that your coworkers are giving you the cold shoulder, warm things up by making a kind gesture. If certain officemates have been especially helpful, give them a small gift of thanks. If you've had to keep people waiting, send an interoffice e-mail showing your gratitude. Men on the most part will be less bothersome. (This is not because they don't feel resentment but because men tend to get weak in the knees when it comes to dealing with female issues. Just mention the words *period* or *cramp* to a guy, and he'll buckle to the floor like a lassoed rodeo calf.) Remember that your coworkers may have to exert some extra effort because you pump, and they don't have a beautiful baby at home to make it all worthwhile. What they can have, however, is a box of chocolates or a fragrant scented candle.

Dress to Express

Getting dressed for work after having a baby can be torture. You've spent the last few months hanging around the house in dirty sweatpants and open blouses. But unless you work at home, you'll be forced to go back to the office and wear appropriate business attire once again. Assuming that you've yet to get back into your prepregnancy shape, you have to buy a whole new wardrobe complete with wider waistbands, looser jackets, and larger-sized pantyhose.

Even if you did manage to shed your baby weight, you're still carrying around two casaba melons where your breasts used to be. This can make buttoning up a shirt rather difficult. And those casabas can leak at the most inopportune moments. That's why, when dressing to express, it's best to stick with clothing that's specifically made for nursing mothers. They make whipping out a booby a breeze and tend to be looser fitting around the bust line so they can house your humongous hooters. When choosing a fabric to minimize the leakage look, go for darker colors, lots of prints, and anything that won't change color much when it's wet.

To avert the eye from your enormous bust line, wear scoop necks instead of boat necks or high-neck shirts. Blazers are great for camouflaging bulging bosoms, as are button-down shirts and anything with vertical pin stripes. Just steer clear of plunging V-necks that look like a giant arrow pointing directly to your abyss of a cleavage. Don't forget to wear accessories like long scarves or long necklaces that give the illusion of an elongated torso, which in turn gives you better proportions.

Yes, dressing for the office can definitely be a challenge when you haven't lost your baby weight and are sporting bowling balls for boobs. But after a few months of nursing, your hormones will settle down, your bust line will shrink, and the leaks will be less frequent. Then the only dressing stress you'll have is squeezing on those damn pantyhose, which are hell to wear no matter your size.

I Want My Mommy

Working moms be warned! At about three months of age, your baby may do something so shocking that you'll rethink your decision to go back to work. No, he won't get a high-powered job that draws a larger salary than your own. What he may do, however, is refuse to take a bottle. When this happens, it will be impossible to concentrate at work since you imagine that your baby is shriveling up like one of those dying pod people in *Cocoon*.

Once babies reach the tender age of three months, they become more aware of their surroundings. They get startled by sounds they never noticed before and look at the world with a whole new fascination. With this sudden awareness comes the realization that it's not their loving mommy who's giving them milk but an imposter otherwise known as Mrs. Doris at Sunshine Day Care.

In the past, your baby would have sucked away happily on his bottle, not caring whose was the hand that fed him. But now he wants only the hand that belongs to you. When it's not, your baby may arch his back, turn his head, and cry in despair as if the caregiver was feeding him a bottle of pomegranate juice. (I know that stuff's all the rage, but man, I think it tastes nasty!)

If this scenario is playing out in your home, relax! This, like all the other upcoming stress-ful stages that your baby will travel through, is only temporary. Assuming that your pediatrician gives your baby the stamp of approval, you need not worry. In fact, worrying only makes matters worse. That's because babies are like little Gei-ger counters. They can pick up on all kinds of disturbances, from your feeding frustrations to the anger you feel when *All My Children* is inter-rupted because of some stupid car chase that the networks feel warrants hours of live coverage.

If your baby is suddenly just saying "no" to a bottle, try the following ideas:

- **Change bottles and nipples.** Some nip-ples may feel more comfortable in your baby's mouth. Babies tend to prefer the nipple size that most closely resembles yours. If they're long, get longer nipples, and if they're short, get the shorter vari-ety. Sometimes caregivers have better suc-cess using spoons, droppers, or even straws than bottles.

- **Change positions.** Try having your care-giver feed your baby close to her chest to mimic the way you do when you nurse. If this doesn't work, try the total opposite approach and have the caregiver give him the bottle from a less intimate position.

- **Don't have the caregiver set herself up for failure by waiting to feed your baby until he's really hungry.** As any waitress will tell you, people get cranky when they need to be fed.

Can't Do It All

Going to the office was hard enough work before you had a baby. You had to wake up early, fight traffic, and ride a crowded elevator while looking up at the numbers so as not to make eye contact with anybody. After putting in a hard day, you then had to run errands on the way home, cook all the meals, and do housework at night and on weekends. On top of all that, you now have all the additional chores of motherhood to take care of as well. It seems that when you go forth and multiply, so does your endless to-do list.

That's why, as embarrassed as you are to admit it and would never say it aloud, a part of you misses the old days before you had a baby. You long for the time when you actually had a moment to yourself. You remember when your husband didn't bug you so much and you actually *wanted* to have sex with him. As much as you hate feeling this way, you feel trapped in your new life.

If this is your mindset, I want to let you in on an unspoken secret of motherhood. At times, every woman feels this way. Being a mother is an endless amount of hard and exhausting work. Feeling resentful and trapped is perfectly normal, but it's rarely talked about even among the closest of friends. It doesn't mean that you're a bad mom. It only means that you're human.

That's why it's crucial to take breaks when you can and let people help you. Taking time to unwind and be alone is not selfish; it's crucial. You can't be a good mom when you're running on empty and have a bad mindset. To help get this important time, it's best to do the things you have to do in the most productive way possible.

One way to do this is to make a list of everything you have to do. In the old days, before morning sickness and mucus plugs, you could get by with a mental to-do list, but now that you've had a baby, your brain cells are working overtime just to keep up. They have to remember how many clean diapers you have left, when the last time was that you fed the baby, and when his last nap was, all while still holding on to vital information like the lyrics to classic Beatles songs and the names of your family members.

During this harried time, it's important to get organized. If you were lucky and had the nesting instinct during your last month of pregnancy, your home may already be as organized as Martha Stewart's craft drawer. If it isn't, go through your closets and throw away, donate, or sell any needless clutter. Then, make sure that everything that remains has a place—and no, thrown on top of the dining-room table is not a "place."

Time management is also crucial, so minimize the workload. Wear your hair in a sleek ponytail instead of having to spend time blowing it dry every morning. Do as many errands as you can online. Get clothing made out of stain-resistant fabric that doesn't need ironing. Buy a slow cooker and throw all your dinner fixings in there in the morning so you can be greeted by a healthy meal at night.

And finally, get as many things done as you can the night before. This includes picking out your next day's outfit, cleaning your breast pump so it's ready in the morning, putting the next day's bottles in the fridge to thaw, and packing your lunch. As you know, mornings can be as chaotic as a Star Trek convention on free Tribble day, so preparation is the key.

With your mornings more relaxed, you'll have time for a feeding before you leave for the office. That way your baby will be full and content before you leave, you'll have longer to work before you need to pump, and your boobs will be emptier so they won't leak during your 10 A.M. client meeting.

Even with all these tips, there'll still be plenty to do. But the more you plan and organize, the easier life will become, and the more free time you'll have. No, you won't yet be bored. Being bored is a luxury that's still a few years away. But you may at least have an hour to yourself to go for a long walk or meet a friend for coffee. It is a terrible thing to have a beautiful baby and be too stressed out and overwhelmed to enjoy him.

Helping Hand

It was only a few generations ago that women didn't have problems juggling both work and baby. That's because for the most part, women didn't work. Instead, the parental roles were clearly defined. Men went out in the workforce and earned the daily bread while women stayed home with the family and turned that bread into tasty sandwiches.

But today women dominate the workforce like never before. So instead of staying in the kitchen, we're now in the corporate world, and we need help getting everything done. If you played your cards right when you were dating, you only went out with kind, loving men who enjoyed long walks on the beach and mopping floors. These are the men who don't mind pitching in with housework and being a part of a family-raising team. But if you were like most of us young, single women, you were drawn to iron men instead of men who could iron, and you're now paying the price by having to do more than your fair share of the household duties.

I don't know how it happened. How, even after women entered the workforce, we're still expected to do most all of the household chores.

Somehow men feel entitled to sit on their asses all weekend watching an endless array of sports while we women run around doing the cooking, cleaning, and errands, and changing poopy diapers. Maybe it's just engrained in the male DNA, along with a bad sense of direction and an inability to remember where they left their wallets. Whatever it is, it's a mystery that's worth solving.

Before you explode with the overwhelming resentment you feel toward your spouse, talk to him. Find a quiet moment when the baby's asleep and the television is off, and let your husband know how you feel in a calm, nonconfrontational manner. Might I also recommend that you don't start off with a statement like, "You don't do enough around the house," but rather, "I'm feeling overwhelmed and I'd really like your help." Hopefully your husband will realize just how unfairly the housework is divided and agree to lend a hand. Then make a list of the things that need to get done on a regular basis and negotiate who does what. Tell him that if he does *A, B,* and *C,* you'll continue to do *S, E,* and *X.*

But please bear one thing in mind. If your partner does take on a certain task, try your dingdong best not to criticize the way he does it. If he folds the towels in half rather than in thirds, so be it. If he loads the dishwasher with the utensils pointing up instead of down, look the other way. As long as his method doesn't hurt or destroy, leave it alone and just be grateful that you don't have to do it yourself. Having a kid means letting go of the strong need to control. Also, when it comes to housework, focus on the important tasks and let others, like washing windows and ironing sheets, go.

If you have older children, have them pitch in as well. Assign them age-appropriate tasks to do around the house. Not only will this make them feel like an integral part of the family, but it will teach them responsibility and how to take care of the things they have. Believe me, it won't do your kids any good to do everything for them. If you do, they'll grow up, get married, and won't have a clue how to take care of their homes. Instead, they'll sit on their asses all weekend watching an endless array of sports while their spouses take care of everything. Hey, I think I may have solved this mystery after all!

Chapter 6

Older and Wearier!

Your little newborn is no longer new. He's had time—and plenty of hearty breast milk—to make him grow big and strong. You look at your child and can't believe he was ever small enough to fit into the outfit he wore when you brought him home from the hospital. Not only does he look different, he acts differently, too. Just when you finally figure out how to get your kid to fall asleep, your trick doesn't work any more. And when you do that thing that always made him laugh, he now just stares at you with a blank look. There is never a dull moment in parenting because you're constantly relearning how to do it. And nursing is no exception to that rule.

You think back on all the struggles you had in order to get your baby to latch on correctly. How many times it took you to pump without pain. Or to forgive your husband when he was alone with your kid and wasted all those bottles of precious pumped milk trying to calm him down, knowing full well that he wasn't hungry. (Actually, I've yet to let that one go.)

So enjoy the miracles that your child performs on a day-to-day basis. Take plenty of pictures and write it all down in his baby book. Your precious bundle of love is growing faster and learning more than he will in any other year of his life. While he's performing these amazing feats, he's bound to cause some frustrations along the way, like the ones that you'll read about in this chapter. But forgive him for misbehaving. Until he's old enough to learn what a time-out is, you'll just have to deal.

Too Busy to Eat

Ah, the good ol' days when you would put your babe to your breast and have a beautiful Hallmark moment. Your newborn would suckle away happily with that "I could do this all day" kind of glow. But now that your baby is older and has discovered the wonderful world around him, his appointment book is full. He has shapes to observe, fans to watch, and a thumb to find. He's way too busy to squeeze in a meal. When you force the issue, he twists and turns and pushes you away like a gay man getting a lap dance. What's a desperate mother to do?

First of all, relax. It's very common for a baby to lose interest in nursing as the months go by. One reason for this new behavior is that his vision is getting better. Before, all he could see was black-and-white blurs. Now he sees the world in its full Technicolor glory, and, as anyone who's witnessed that amazing scene when Dorothy walks into Munchkin Land knows, it's an awe-inspiring transition.

The world also sounds more interesting than it did before. Now, when your baby hears the phone ring or the "clickity click" sound of the dog's nails on the hardwood floor, it's as fascinating to him as the "Attention Kmart shoppers" announcement is to you. When your baby hears a noise as he's nursing, he'll instantly let go of your nipple and turn toward the sound. You'll try to get him interested again but, as with you and the Kmart announcement, he now has a one-track mind.

Even though it's a struggle to nurse your baby now that he's older, there are some ways to minimize the battle:

- **Nurse in a dark, quiet room.** Dim the lights, turn off the distant radio or television, and get down to business.
- **If you're out in public, use a sling to nurse.** Your baby will be very relaxed, and the high walls on the sling will act like horse blinders to minimize the distractions. Even if your baby does turn his head to see what's going on, he'll quickly learn that his efforts don't amount to squat.
- **Don't delay feeding times.** Oddly enough, when babies get too hungry, they resist nursing entirely. It's the same oddity as when they get so overtired they refuse to go to sleep. Aren't kids whacky?

Like most other phases that your baby goes through, he'll tend to pass through this one rather quickly as well. I guarantee that the person who made up the saying "The only thing constant is change" was the parent of a nursing baby. In the meantime, you may have to suffer through less-effective nursing sessions more often, at least

"Once my baby learned to sit up, he only wanted to nurse in that position. My boobs were big, but not big enough to be able to make that ninety-degree turn to fit inside his mouth."

—Jeanie

until your little peanut grows tired of observing the plant on your coffee table or listening to the sound of the mailman coming to the door. By that time, however, your little one will develop the ability to sit up, and nursing will become even more difficult. Sitting up is an amazing feat for a baby, and it warrants excitement equal to what you'd feel if you were suddenly able to fly.

During this time, you shouldn't think that your baby's lack of interest in breastfeeding is his way of telling you that he has the desire to wean. It's quite unusual for an infant to choose to wean. More often than not, he's just grown more interested in the world around him.

As with everything else in nursing, and in mommy-dom, the answer is to just relax. Even though your kid gets distracted, by the end of the day, he really is eating enough food. Unless your doctor has told you that your baby isn't gaining weight at a healthy rate, it's safe to assume that he'll eat when he needs to eat. Right now he's just busy discovering the world. You may know how he feels if you're one of those lucky women who can be so busy they're not interested in food. Me, I've yet to find anything more interesting than a New York cheesecake!

Don't Bite the Breast That Feeds You

Does your kid chew your nipple like a piece of Juicy Fruit? Is he causing you to swear more than a Def Comedy Jam when it's feeding time? Then you've entered the not-so-wonderful world of mothers who suffer the slings and arrows of outrageous torture every time they feed their teething kids.

Babies get teeth at various times. Some may get them a few weeks after delivery, others after a year. But sooner or later, your baby will grow some enamel torture devices that turn his mouth into public enemy number one. It's as if your kid was cutting Ginzu knives. To make matters worse, when your baby teethes, his natural instinct is to bite down hard to relieve the pain. He'll bite on anything he comes in contact with. Your finger. The dog's tail. Whatever can fit inside his mouth. And as you know, your nipples are one of the things that are most commonly in there.

Although your baby is the biter, you may play a part in the problem. Chances are, the first time your baby bit down on your nipple, you made the horrible, yet natural, mistake of being startled and yelping, "Ouch!" That no doubt tickled your baby's fancy, leading him to bite you like a pit bull during every feeding. Then, after each attack, you yanked him off your chest like an itchy sweater. That of course, only led to more pain, suffering, and bloody nipples.

That's why, if your wee one has yet to take his first bite, you should nip the behavior in the bud. The very first time he clamps down, shout, "No!" If you're lucky, this should scare the crap out of him, a good thing if he's suffering from constipation.

If you've already set up the pattern of biting, it doesn't mean that you can't put an end to it. I know your first instinct is to talk to your child in a placating voice and say, "You're hurting Mommy, and I'd like you to stop now." Go ahead and see how far you get. While you're at it, you may as well tell him to sleep through the night and clean his room. After you exhaust your willingness to try the diplomacy method, try some of these techniques:

- Keep your index finger close to his mouth while nursing. This is a handy tool you can use to break the seal as soon as he begins to bite. Just put it between his mouth and your breast and pop him off you like an easy-open lid.
- Push your baby into your breast. That will quickly make him open his mouth and pull away since he won't be able to breathe through his nose. Not only will this stop further damage to your already used and abused nipple, but it will fortify the notion that if your baby bites, something bad will happen.
- Safely detach your baby as soon as he bites and put him in a position that he doesn't favor, like on his stomach or flat on his back. Again, this will enforce the notion that biting has its consequences.

Often times, babies start nipping after their bellies are full and they're ready for the entertainment portion of the evening. That's all the more reason for pulling him off once he bites so that he'll associate biting with the end of the nursing session.

Once you've removed your baby and feeding time is over, give him something more productive to deal with teething pain than your chest area. Offer him a teether or a frozen washcloth (or frozen bagel or frozen banana, if he's old enough for solid food). Soon he'll learn that your teet is not a toy.

I'm Low on Milk

Every new mother has the same worries. She worries that she won't be a good parent. She worries she'll never lose her baby weight and spend the rest of her life wearing overalls. But by far the biggest concern for a nursing mother is that she's not producing enough milk. Fortunately, after a few weeks when she sees her baby's chubby cheeks and pudgy toes, that worry fades away.

But then after a few months, she'll notice that her once Hummer-sized hooters have been reduced to the size of Mini Coopers, and her worries return. Where did all her milk go? And why is her nursing bra suddenly loose? Once again, I must advise you to relax. Stress only makes matters worse, and if you're an emotional eater, this will only make giving up those overalls more difficult. It's perfectly normal for your breasts to deflate to a fairly normal size after a couple of months of regular nursing.

You see, after delivery, your breasts are like little Jewish mothers: They make way too much for your bubalah to drink. If you think about it, you'll realize that your breasts can't read ultrasounds. They don't know for sure how many children you're going to have, and they need to be prepared. After several weeks of going overboard on production, your milk supply is reduced, and your breasts become less full. But that doesn't mean that you're running low on milk. All it means is that your body is adjusting to the amount of milk it needs to produce in order to feed your bubalah.

Sometimes this change happens so slowly that mothers aren't even aware it's happened until they notice some give in the bra region. Others only notice that they're leaking less when their less full breasts don't spring as many leaks. But other times the change happens quickly, leading new mothers to panic that the well has run dry, which leads to supplementing with formula, which leads to weaning.

So stop worrying, and realize that your smaller breasts are still keeping up with your baby's needs. Okay, I guess it *is* a mother's job to worry, so you can worry a little if you must. But then sit back and enjoy the fact that you can button your shirt without the top buttons flying across the room, and you can have sex without squirting your lover in the eye.

A Good Solid Meal

As your baby grows, so do his nutritional needs. At first, your little one was content eating only from the dairy food group. But somewhere between the ages of four and six months, his palate will become more sophisticated, and he'll take an interest in the food that's on your plate. He'll watch you gobble down your fries with the same thrill as a roaring game of peek-a-boo. (Hey, that's pretty exciting stuff for a baby.) It's at this time you'll realize that your baby isn't a baby anymore and that he may be ready to eat solid foods.

This is an exciting period for parents. Not only is this a stepping stone in your baby's development, but, yippee for you, you get to do a new activity during the day. By now, you've read *Pat the Bunny* a million times and sang "You Are My Sunshine" a million more. The thought of doing something new is as exciting to you as that roaring game of peek-a-boo. (Hey, you're exhausted and can't handle much more excitement than that anyway.) Talk to your pediatrician, and if he gives you the go ahead, go to the market and get some baby food.

Your baby's first gourmet meal of choice will no doubt be baby rice cereal with expressed breast milk. You'll put the spoon to his mouth and expect him to wolf it down like a box of Double Stuf Oreos, but chances are he'll end up getting more of it *on* him than *in* him. As you can imagine, eating from a spoon is a lot different than drinking from a nipple, and it will take some time for him to conquer this feat. If you have a problem eating rice with chopsticks, you'll understand just where he's coming from. But with a little practice, it shouldn't take long before eats more than he drops, which is more than you can say about the chopsticks.

While your baby is learning, it's important to continue nursing as well as that's where your child will still get most of his nutritional needs met. It's a good idea to nurse for a few minutes before you begin feeding solids. If your baby is overly hungry, he's more likely to turn a meal into a meltdown. Once he's finished eating the cereal, you can then top him off with more breast milk until he's full.

As the weeks go by, you'll continue to introduce a variety of new foods, from vegetables to fruits to meats. Your pediatrician should give you a breakdown of which foods to introduce in which order and which items to avoid during the first year (such as honey and highly allergenic foods). As your baby eats more and more, you may find that you'll smile more and more, too. That's because solids tend to satisfy your kid longer than breast milk alone, which means that he can last longer between feedings. Also, with a full belly at bedtime, he'll probably sleep for longer stretches as well. As you know, when baby sleeps better, you sleep better, too. And that's the greatest gift a new mother can receive . . . next to a good hemorrhoid pillow, of course.

Dinner and a Show

There's no doubt about it. Kids are cutie pies. But what they have in looks, they lack in social graces. They scream in public, drool uncontrollably, and crap all over themselves. And when they nurse, these little love bugs commit numerous nursing faux pas that are frowned upon by members of high society.

The most upsetting nursing no-no is what your baby does with his spare hand when you breastfeed. Sure, one of his hands is kept safely in lockdown mode, but the other is free to roam about and explore his surroundings. This hand twiddles your nipple, pinches your underarm, scratches your chest, and performs other acts of battery that could get him five to ten in a state penitentiary.

Even worse is when you're in public and these little no-no's become giant nightmares, especially when your little one commits the heinous act of lifting up your shirt à la Drew Barrymore on Letterman. You panic, which makes him chuckle, which in turn makes him want to perform this little burlesque routine whenever there's an audience to enjoy it.

Once your baby gets older and is able to move around at will, he may get bored with the one standard nursing position he's been doing all of his young life and want to spice things up a bit. He'll want to try breastfeed while sitting up, lying on the floor, or contorting into some position that can only be achieved by someone whose bones have not yet fused. You'll try to appease him, but alas, your breasts aren't large enough to manage some of those maneuvers.

"I'm so used to my daughter groping and fondling me every
time she nurses that I'm not even aware she's doing it.
I only notice it when I'm in a public place and everyone
starts staring at me. I know I should be embarrassed,
but it's the closest I'll ever be to feeling like a celebrity."

—Georgia

If your baby is starting to "play with his food,"
it's time to do something about it. Nursing is
enough of an effort without adding these types of
irritations, embarrassments, and torn ligaments
to the mix. Here are some suggestions on how to
get your kid back in the nursing saddle again:

- **Give your child something to hold on to.** Let him play with a toy instead of your upper body.
- **Give your child something interesting to look at.** Make a colorful nursing necklace out of kitchen twine and beads or plastic objects.
- **Distract him by singing a song or telling him a story.** Be sure to make lots of facial expressions so that you'll hold his interest instead of him holding your nipple.

- **Give him alternatives.** If he has a specific need to do with his hand, such as stroke your hair, offer a suitable replacement like a silky pillow.
- **Stop the action.** If your child likes to lift up your shirt every time he takes a swig, pull it back tightly back so it'll stay in place. After several attempts, he'll get bored trying. Or you can commit to wearing only a nursing shirt in public so that your baby can't do his burlesque routine.
- **Head him off at the pass.** If your baby likes to play with your non-nursing breast when he eats, don't unhook that side of your bra. That way, he's not able to get to the goods.
- **Break the suction every time he does a behavior that you don't like and say "no."** It won't take long for him to realize that actions have their consequences. This is an important life lesson and one to know when he starts drawing on walls or gets married and forgets to remove the receipt from the strip club from his back pocket.

Pre-Conception

Now that your baby's getting older, there's another important issue to discuss. You may have heard the rumor that as long as you continue to nurse, you don't have to worry about using birth control. Well, I'm here to tell you that rumor is undeniably false. If it were true, I wouldn't be here today, and you'd have just plopped down good money for a blank book since I wouldn't have been around to write it. You see, my mother conceived me when my sister was only three months old. She, too, believed those rumors and thought that as long as she nursed, she'd be okay. Sucker.

But (and I say this in the most conservative, "Don't sue me if it's not true in your case" kind of way), you will have a far less chance of conceiving if you breastfeed than if you don't because nursing impedes ovulation. This is especially true during the first three months, when you're nursing round the clock. It's especially true under certain conditions, such as the following:

- You breastfeed on demand, both day and night.
- You don't use any bottles or pacifiers. (Again, pacifiers may reduce SIDS, so

speak with your pediatrician about what's best for you and your situation.)
- Your baby is not eating solid foods.
- You are not pumping.
- You do not have a period.
- You're too exhausted to have sex . . . just kidding, but who the heck wants to have sex during those first few months anyway!

In general, the more you nurse, the more effective nursing is at preventing pregnancy. But once your baby is able to last longer between feedings and is sleeping better at night, the effectiveness of nursing as a form of birth control starts to decrease. To add even more fertile bang for the buck, once your baby becomes less demanding, your husband usually becomes even more so . . . in bed, that is. You have to realize that his sex drive has been drastically denied these past few months (even longer if you count the last month of pregnancy. when the only things you wanted inside of you were your doctor's hands to see if you'd started dilating). Now that you have more energy, your husband's engine is back in high gear.

There is no typical time when you can expect to get your period again. Some women start up just a few months after delivery, while others might not start for a year. But whenever Aunt Flo does come a-calling once again, you can expect her visit to be quite upsetting. Here your lochia has finally stopped flowing, your privates have recovered from delivery, and you're able to go to the bathroom without craving anti-anxiety medication. After all that torture, the last thing you want to deal with so soon is cramping and PMS. It's enough to make you want a career as a surrogate so you won't have to deal with your period ever again.

That's why it's important to use some method of birth control if you don't want to have two rug rats in diapers. If you're nursing, the pill isn't your best choice because it contains hormones that can reduce your milk supply. A diaphragm is a good choice, but if you used a diaphragm before, you'll need to have it checked out by your gynecologist to see if it still fits. You can also use the rhythm method, which is basically taking the stuff you learned about ovulation and reversing it so you only have sex during low-risk times.

So, if you're not ready to give your baby a sibling, you may need more than just nursing to stop yourself from going forth and multiplying. Talk to your doctor and see which method of birth control is best for you. Or let your husband be in charge of contraception and use a condom. Lord knows there's enough on your plate to deal with right now, and since he didn't have any labor pains, lochia, painful delivery, or traumatic poops, it really is his turn to make a sacrifice.

Chapter 7

You're a Weaner!

Every woman has a different experience when it comes to breastfeeding. Some find it to be a tender and loving way to bond with their babies like no one else on the planet can. Others find it to be something to endure, like chronic back pain or always choosing the slowest line at the supermarket, but they do it anyway in order to give their babies the very best they can. No matter whether you savor the experience or sour on it, there will come a time when you call it quits and put your overworked boobies up on the high shelf, along with your high school tube tops and midriff-revealing tees.

Just as every woman has a different experience when it comes to breastfeeding, each will have a different experience of weaning, too. That's because no two babies are alike, and they all take to weaning differently. Some kids don't have much trouble giving up the breast; others become so addicted you'll wish you could send them to the Betty Ford clinic.

While several factors come into play when determining the ease of your weaning experience, there is one aspect to it that's universal: You will have far greater success at weaning if you are strongly committed to doing it. If you're on the fence about whether it's the right time to start, or whether you're doing it for the right reason, then don't even try. Wait until you're convinced that getting your babe off your boob is the right choice for you. Babies have the ability to manipulate you like Play-Doh, so if you're feeling guilty or are wishy-washy on the subject, you can expect more setbacks and more frustrations.

Once you have the right mindset, weaning will be a relative breeze (relative to other challenges you face, like making your baby sleep better or getting your husband to pick up after himself). In hopes of getting the weaning ball rolling, here are some valuable tips you should know about before you pull the plug on your milk supply.

All the Cool Moms Are Doing It

Sure, the medical community advises that you wait six months before you wean, but they also advise you to stay out of the sun and eat five servings of fruits and veggies a day, and you don't take their advice about that stuff either. When it comes to weaning, you should do what works best for you in your own situation. If you can breastfeed for six months, fine. If you can go so long that your kid has to take out his retainer in order to nurse, that's fine too. (Okay, it's a bit odd, but I'm trying remain nonjudgmental here.) But if, for whatever reason, you want or need to stop nursing before six months are through, there is no reason to feel guilty about your decision or to think that you're a bad mother. Million of mothers wean their babies long before that time, and their kids still thrive just the same. So if you want to hop on the cool-mom bandwagon with all the other early weaners, hop away. In fact, here are some of the times babies are most commonly weaned before that half-birthday hallmark:

After the first few weeks of nursing: Many new moms want to give nursing a try, but they find it too frustrating and painful to continue. Also, having a newborn can often be so overwhelming and exhausting that nursing is the first item of stress to go.

When it's time to go back to work: No matter how big your boobs are, they're not able to make the commute from your office to your baby, and some moms don't have the desire to pump.

When your baby starts getting teeth: Whoever said, "The first cut is the deepest" must have been referring to the pain of those razor-sharp teeth on her delicate nipples. True, if you had the gumption, you could work through this stage and dissuade your baby from biting. (See "Don't Bite the Breast That Feeds You, on page 168.) But if you're looking for a reason to stop nursing, teething could just be the straw that broke the camel's back, or in this case, your areola.

A painful nursing ailment such as mastitis or a breast infection: Of course, you can't wean while you're healing, but once your breasts are back on their feet, many women start the weaning process so that they'll never have to go through that kind of trauma again.

Baby's lack of interest in nursing: Sure, that lack could easily be caused by his increased interest in other things, or maybe it's because of the different taste in your milk due to hormonal changes or last night's kung pao chicken. But if you're losing interest in nursing as well, this will certainly be as good an excuse as any to start the weaning process.

When the stick turns blue: Although many pregnant women can handle breastfeeding one child while suffering through morning sickness with another, others can't. If you're expecting, you may also expect that your baby's days of nursing are numbered.

As you can see, there are many valid reasons to stop nursing. So if you're one of the millions of mothers who stops before her baby is six months old, don't despair. Realize that any amount of breast milk you were able to give your baby has been good. There are many more important things to feel guilty about, about like the time you cut his nails so short that they bled.

The Chest Alternative

Before you start denying your baby access to your boobies, you have to teach him how to drink from something other than yourself. If you were worried about nipple confusion or have never been away from your baby very long, he may not have any experience using a bottle. When teaching your baby how to use a bottle, it's best to give that assignment to someone other than yourself. Your baby knows that you have his favorite beverage on hand (or in chest), and he may not be happy if you offer him a substitute.

Don't expect your baby to make the transition from breast to bottle right away. Chances are good that he'll resist it and spit it out like a bad clam. As you can imagine, the way your baby sucks from a bottle is much different than how he latches on to you. (See "Nip/Stuck" on page 112.) If your baby is rejecting the bottle more than the daytime Emmys rejected Susan Lucci, experiment with different shapes of bottles or nipples. America is the land of the plenty. If they can make twelve varieties of bologna, you can bet they make a wide selection of bottles and nipples to choose from as well.

If your baby is adamant about his rejection of the bottle, offer him a sippy cup with a straw, if he's old enough to manage it. Or you can try a regular sippy cup that's held like a bottle and needs to be inverted to operate. You can also find sippy cup tops that are used on standard-size bottles. Using a sippy cup can often make for an easier transition from boob to bottle. For some reason, little tykes are interested in the sippy cup. Perhaps it makes them more feel more grown up, not unlike how that cigarette did when you were in junior high.

There's another kink lying ahead in the pre-weaning system. You have to decide what kind of beverage to put inside the cup or bottle. One option, of course, is expressed breast milk, a popular choice among mothers who are returning to work. Another option is formula. If your little tax deduction is older than a year, you can go directly to whole cow's milk, but you should choose one that's free of the artificial growth hormone BGH unless you want your little girl to need tampons when she's nine. While it may not be proven that there's a connection between eating hormone-ridden food and early puberty, why take a chance? *Your* menstrual cycles wreak enough havoc on the household already.

So no matter whether you go with a bottle or a cup, formula or milk, just be sure that your baby is comfortable drinking from something other than your chest before you even think about starting the weaning process. Once your baby is comfortable with your choices, you're "weady to wean"!

Pick a Date

Picking a date to start weaning is very similar to picking a date to start a diet. You don't want to set yourself up for failure by starting a diet near Valentine's Day, when heart-shaped boxes line the store shelves. Likewise, there are certain times when you don't want to start weaning your baby.

So when is the perfect time to wean? There is none. Some prefer to start when their babies are younger and more malleable. They haven't had time to build up a strong preference or strong enough lung capacity to throw a tantrum when they don't get what they want. Other parents wait until their kids are older and their instinct to suck isn't as strong. They also know that once solids foods are introduced, their babies will get more nourishment from other sources than just a steady stream of breast milk.

No matter how old your child is when weaning begins, it may be a rough road ahead. That's why it's important to pick a time to start that's devoid of any big emotional or physical change. Sure, you can't predict the future, and you don't know if your child is going to get sick or be hurt, but there are predictable periods that cause everyone stress that should be avoided like the plague, or like holiday shopping on Christmas Eve:

During a family trip: Even the most enjoyable vacation goes hand in hand with stress. For you, it's the long lines at the airport or a hotel room that doesn't have a fully stocked mini-bar. For your baby, it's sleeping in a different bed and dealing with a time change. Adding weaning to the mix turns a weekend in paradise into a weekend of hell on Earth.

When your baby starts day care or has a new sitter: Babies are creatures of habit. When you make a change in their routines, it can register as a ten on their internal Richter scales. Adding weaning on top of this situation will create a shockwave that will be heard around your neighborhood.

When you're moving to a new home: Even if you're moving from a dump to a deluxe apartment in the sky, moving is hard. There are boxes to pack, utilities to change, and barking dogs at night that you never heard before because you only saw your house during the day. Weaning is one stress that you can certainly do without.

During the holiday season: Once we were old enough to stop believing in Santa, our holidays became an endless list of gifts to buy, and an endless line at the post office in order to send them. When you add weaning to the mix, I simply say, "Bah humbug!"

Slow and Steady Weans the Race

There are certain things that are best to get over with quickly, like ripping off a bandage or plucking the hairs that grow from your big toe . . . OUCH! But other things, like weaning, are best to do slowly. If you wean too quickly, you can face engorgement problems, breast ailments, and mood swings that rival any you had during pregnancy.

"I had the baby blues after I gave birth and had a tough time for awhile. But it was nothing compared with the blues I felt when I started weaning. One minute I'd be screaming and the next, I'd be really depressed. In the past, I never believed those women who used hormonal changes as a reason to commit a crime, but now I completely understand it."

—Allison

In order to wean slowly, it's important to drop only one feeding at a time. Dropping any more will be hard on both your baby and your body. If you can, choose the feeding that's the least important to your baby in terms of nourishment and bonding. In most instances, that'll be the one during the middle of the day, when your baby has so many other exciting things to do—like watching the cat lick herself.

Once you stop a feeding, it will take your body a few days to cease producing milk during that time. Until then be prepared with ice packs and nursing pads, and if you must, express only as little as you need to make yourself comfortable. While you're giving up feedings, you may experience mood swings, crankiness, or depression as your hormone levels adjust. It will take your body a minimum of three days to get comfortable with a missed feeding, so be sure not to drop any more feeding until that adjustment is made.

After that time period, you can drop another feeding. And so on and so on, until you have no more feedings and your breasts become as dry as Palm Springs. If you'd like, you don't have to give up all your feeding and can elect to keep one or two that you enjoy the most. In most cases, these are the relaxing ones that take place at the beginning and end of each day when your kidlette is all sleepy and delicious. True, you may not have as much milk as you did before, but both you and your bambino can still enjoy the experience.

To make weaning go smoother, avoid trigger points that will make your kid crave the breast more than your old prom date did. For instance, if you always nurse in a certain chair, don't sit in it. If you sing a certain lullaby when you nurse, don't sing it. If your baby has already had a bottle or a snack and still looks at your chest with a gleam in his eye, become a moving target. Offer him a toy or instigate a roaring game of "how big is baby?" If Daddy is home, have him be the playmate since his hairy chest doesn't conjure up the same images of maids a milkin' in your baby's head.

"My toddler would always stare at my chest as if it were full of mac 'n' cheese. I tried to distract him whenever he looked at my breasts and wore high-necked shirts so he couldn't get his hands on me. I realized I was treating my son like I was my husband whenever he wanted sex."

—Annie

Like any habit, it will take some time to quit nursing. But if you do it slowly, your kid's cravings should diminish along with your milk supply and your mood swings. Yes, I know you've heard stories of women who rubbed unsweetened cocoa powder or apple cider vinegar on their nipples in an attempt to get their kids to stop nursing fast. Or about the mothers who went away on vacation for a week all by themselves and returned to a totally weaned kid. But when it comes to weaning, slow and steady really does win the race. Maybe you don't get to spend seven days on a sandy beach with a mai tai in your hand, but it's still your best bet.

Alternative

Another excellent way to wean is to lessen the amount of breast milk given at each feeding. Take your baby off your boob before he empties it. Then offer milk from the bottle or sippy cup until he's full. As the days go by, give him less and less until your breasts are empty. Weaning in this manner provides less engorgement and hormone fluxes, too. What it doesn't provide however, is that four- to five-hour stretch of time that you can be away from your baby.

Don't Touch My Titties!

Weaning is a process. It takes time, patience, and a lot of trying moments. And you don't want anything to slow down this process, like having let down occur. That's why, when you start weaning, it's common to treat your breasts like a classic Disney film and lock them away in the vault until it's time to bring them out again. You know that any stimulation can cause this unwanted let down and signal your body that it still needs to produce milk. At a moment's notice, don't be surprised if you do one or more of the following behaviors:

- You instinctually bite your lovers' hand if it comes anywhere near your chest.
- You don't let your breasts face the stream of warm water in the shower.
- You stop watching any television show that has a baby in it on the remote chance that he will cry.
- You refuse to give yourself your monthly breast exam.
- You let your breasts air dry instead of rubbing them with a towel after you bathe.
- You give your kid anything he wants so that he won't start fussing. In fact, you do so to every kid in the neighborhood.
- You tell your husband you've got some sort of discharge and can't have sex until further notice. Hearing the word *discharge* will kill any man's mood.

Withdrawal Symptoms

We all know how hard it is to kick a habit. Whether it's reality television, trashy magazines, or creamy onion dip, giving up something we love can be a horrendous, life-altering experience. If quitting is hard for us grown people, just imagine how terrorizing it can be to an itty-bitty person who freaks out if we simply leave the room for a moment. Weaning is difficult because nursing provides your little one with far more than just a belly full of grub. It also gives him a great deal of comfort. When you nurse your baby in your arms, you're not only feeding his body, you're feeding his spirit as well. That's why when you start to wean, there are plenty of times that your baby wants your boob, even when he's not hungry.

One of these times is when your baby is sick. Whether he's suffering from the misery of the sniffles or the perils of the flu, your baby will want to be attached to your breast like a tassel on a Vegas showgirl. In this case, nursing not only provides your baby comfort but also much-needed antibodies to help him fight off the illness. As you can imagine, it'll be hard for your baby to get over a habit when he's under the weather.

The boob also helps soothe the savage beast, or in this case, the "tantruming toddler." As you may have experienced, your growing child is bombarded with emotions he doesn't quite understand and can struggle with the emotional overload. When this happens, nursing your baby is like pressing the reset button on your garbage disposal. It instantly calms your baby down.

Your baby also wants the boob when he's having trouble sleeping. Nursing is like baby Ambien and gets your child to sleep faster than you can say *Goodnight Moon*. Once you take away the breast, your baby may have a hard time falling to sleep if he's used to doing so while he nurses. If you have yet to teach your baby to fall asleep on his own, do yourself a favor and spend a couple of weeks dealing with this issue before you even think about weaning. Taking away his warm milk at bedtime *and* making him learn how to fall asleep on his own is enough to make him go into full-fledged detox mode.

So if your baby is having trouble weaning during these or other emotionally trying times, offer plenty of cuddles and distraction. If times get too hard, go ahead and nurse until the problem is over and he's back to himself again. Setbacks happen in all aspects of baby learning, from weaning to potty training. But somehow we all learned how to give up the boob and not urinate at will, so moms must be doing something right!

Conclusion

The Breast Is Back!

Not long after your baby suckles his last meal from your mammaries, you'll start to notice some changes. For one, you'll find that you're not so ravenously thirsty and don't have the constant need to down Lake Tahoe. You'll find that you're not so hungry either and can actually go to a restaurant without devouring your basket of bread, and your neighbor's, before your meal even arrives.

Because your eating habits change, you may finally drop some of the weight you couldn't drop before and find that your clothes are getting looser. Unfortunately, so is your bra. Not only does weaning quickly return your breasts to their pre-pregnancy cup size, it may take it one step further and returns them to your pre-*pubescent* cup size.

You revel in the fact that after months of sharing your body with someone else (maybe even years, if you include your pregnancy), you can finally call your body your own again and do with it as you please. You can freely partake in apple martinis, put the hot sauce back on your chili, and ingest medicine again to relieve your aches and pains. You can also have sex without an extra-strength lubricant or drenching your loved one because you have squirt guns for nipples.

You'll find that your clothing style changes when you wean, too. You can finally put away those stretched-out, stained nursing shirts and go back to wearing clothing without peek-a-boo holes (unless it's a special night and your husband requests that you do). You can wear pants that have button flies instead of drawstring waists and bras with underwire. And you can wear nice underwear again without worry since your periods are back to their predictable twenty-eight day cycle.

Surprisingly enough, for the first time since you peed on an ovulation stick, you find that you're actually thinking about having another kid. Knowing that you have what it takes to nurse a baby and keep him healthy gives you the confidence to do it again. It's like that time you kept that temperamental orchid alive all winter and went out a bought a few more.

Now when you go out in public with your child and watch a new mom struggle to nurse with dignity, you want to tell her it'll all be okay. That soon it *will* get easier and that she too will become one of those moms who can nurse their baby, chat on their cell phone, and butter their roll all at the same time. As you watch her struggle to cover herself with a blanket and grimace in pain when her baby latches on, a part of you will feel relief. You'll glance at your little one sitting happily in his highchair, eating the Cheerios you've scattered on his plate, and you'll be glad that that stage of your life is over.

But surprisingly, you'll also find that a part of you feels sad. For even though nursing brought you an endless stream of challenges and cabbage leaves, leaving you not much time to yourself and straining your marriage to the breaking point, a part of you will always miss it. You'll realize how precious that period of time really was and that you'll never be bonded like that with your baby ever again. No matter how much nursing may have sucked while you were going through it, you'll forget about the sore nipples and breast clogs and the hell you went through with growth spurts and pumping at the office, and you'll remember only the good. And that, my dear mommy friend, is one of the most miraculous things about nursing, and motherhood as a whole. So here's to your hard work, your kind spirit, and your willingness to go through so much to give your baby the very best you can. You are Mommy. Let your beauty shine!

Appendix

Resource Section

In this section, you'll find more resources to help you with your nursing challenges.

Where to Find a Lactation Consultant

If you're having trouble nursing and need help, contact a lactation specialist—stat! You can find one by contacting your birthing hospital, pediatrician, or even by looking in the Yellow Pages. In addition to those resources, here are some other ideas:

La Leche League: This organization started more than fifty years ago when breastfeeding rates dropped 20 percent. Over the years, its members have been instrumental in spreading the word about the benefits of nursing and have provided help to millions of women. For more information, go online to *www.lalecheleague.org*.

The International Lactation Consultation Association (ILAC): This is the professional association for international board-certified lactation consultants, as well as other professional health-care providers who deal with women who nurse. You can find them online at *www.ilac.org*.

Two of the biggest breast-pump manufacturers can help you locate a lactation consultant in your area. Call them at the following toll-free numbers:

Medela: (800) 835-5968
Hollister: (800) 323-8750

How to Take Matters into Your Own Hands

There will be many times when expressing your breast milk by hand can be beneficial. Some of those times include dealing with engorgement, weaning, or getting milk to mix in with your baby's rice cereal. To express milk by hand, follow these steps:

1. Place your thumb on top of your areola and your fingers underneath it at the outer margin.

2. Press back toward your chest and gently squeeze your thumb and fingers together as you pull back out again. Do this rhythmic motion again and again until the milk is expressed.

3. Reposition your fingers so you drain the milk from all the ducts. When finished, do the other side. You can try to milk your breasts for another round if you need additional milk.

Nursing Wear

You just had a baby and are too busy to go shopping. Here are some places to shop for cute nursing clothes without ever leaving your house:

- Motherwear.com: Lots of selection
- Onehotmama.com: Nursing clothes for the clothing conscious
- Babystyle.com: They can be bit pricy, but their clothes are darn cute. They also have a line of transitional clothing, such as lots of elastic and drawstring waistbands.
- Jakeandme.com: Specializes in plus sizes and tall nursing clothing

Where to Donate Your Excess Breast Milk

If you're one of those lucky women who has no problem making milk and have more than enough to go around, consider donating the excess to a hospital NICU near you. They usually arrange for pickup and make the process an easy one. To find a local hospital with babies in need of breast milk, contact the Human Milk Banking Association of North America, online at *www.hmbana.org*.

Sleeping Books

Before you start weaning, make sure your baby can fall asleep without nursing. Here are some good books to help teach your kid to fall asleep on his own:

- *The No-Cry Sleep Solution: Gentle Ways to Help Your Baby Sleep Through the Night,* by Elizabeth Pantley (McGraw-Hill)
- *Healthy Sleep Habits, Happy Child,* by Marc Weissbluth, M.D. (Ballantine Books)
- *Bedtime Sucks,* by me, Joanne Kimes (yes, a shameless plug, but I think it's a darn good book nonetheless) with Kathleen Laccinole (Adams Media)

Index

About the Author

Breastfeeding Sucks is the eighth book in the *Sucks* series. Joanne Kimes has also written for numerous comedy and children's television shows. She and her husband, Jeff, live in Studio City, CA, with their long-weaned daughter, Emily. Visit her at *www.sucksandthecity.com*.

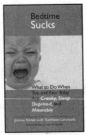
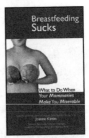
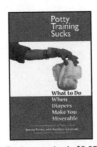
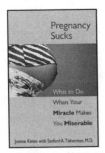
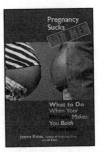